BLACK
and
MINORITY
ETHNIC GROUPS
in
ENGLAND

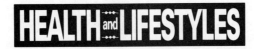

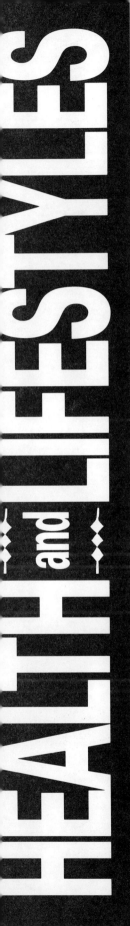

HEALTH and LIFESTYLES

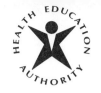

HEALTH EDUCATION AUTHORITY

BLACK
and
MINORITY
ETHNIC GROUPS
in
ENGLAND

This report was written for the Health Education Authority
by Kai Rudat, MORI Health Research Unit.

ISBN 0 7521 0322 9

First published 1994

Health Education Authority
Hamilton House
Mabledon Place
London WC1H 9TX

Typeset by Type Generation Ltd

Printed in Great Britain by BPC Wheatons Ltd, Exeter

Contents

Foreword   vii

Acknowledgements   ix

Introduction   1

1 **Background and methodology**   5
   Background   5
   The qualitative research   6
   Questionnaire development   8
   Main fieldwork   15

2 **Demographic factors**   22
   Age and gender profile   22
   Country of birth   23
   Languages spoken   24
   Languages read   28
   Work status   31
   Education   36
   Housing   38

3 **Perceptions of health**   41
   Health status   41
   Risk factors   47
   Involvement in health-enhancing activities   51

4 **Use of health services**   54
   Registration with a GP   54
   Use of primary care services   55
   Reason for last visit to GP   58
   Physical access to GPs   60
   Appointments and waiting times   61
   Ethnicity of GP   63
   Language of communication   65
   Use of interpreters   66
   Quality of communication   67
   Gender preference for GP   69
   Contact with other members of the primary care team   70
   Use of other health services   71
   Cancer screening   72

5 **Smoking**   78

    Smoking prevalence   78

    Cigarette consumption   81

    Chewing of paan, betel nut, and other substances   82

    Passive smoking   84

    Perceived health effects   88

    Smoking cessation   91

    Smoking cessation attempts amongst current regular smokers   95

    Workplace smoking policy   98

6 **Health promotion**   101

    Health promotion activities   101

    Use of other health information services   113

    Future issues for health promotion   115

References   119

Appendix. Example questionnaire   122

Foreword

The Health Education Authority and the NHS Ethnic Health Unit are working closely together to promote the health of black and minority ethnic groups and both organisations recognise the importance of the provision of information to support others working in this area.

This report makes a major contribution to the range of initiatives for promoting health in black and minority ethnic groups in England which the Health Education Authority has planned as part of a strategy addressing the health needs of these groups.

The Health Education Authority has commissioned two health and lifestyles surveys of these groups. The results from the first of these are reported here. Together the surveys will provide the most important and comprehensive study of knowledge, attitude, behaviour and health status among black and minority ethnic groups in England. No other survey has covered such a wide range of issues pertinent to health promotion on a national scale. It will contribute significantly to identifying the health promotion needs of specific ethnic minority groups.

This report represents a significant first step towards disseminating the results from this pioneering study. The results will help inform the work of the Health Education Authority, the NHS Ethnic Health Unit and other organisations involved in work with these populations at either national or local level. I recommend this report to everyone involved in planning programmes of work to tackle health inequalities and to help meet the Health of the Nation targets.

Michael Chan
Director
NHS Ethnic Health Unit

Acknowledgements

Thanks are due to the many people who contributed to this project. Particular thanks are due to Jeanie McKenzie, Rosemary Pope and Jacky Chambers who were involved in the early stages of this work and have since left the HEA. More recently, major contributions have been made by the current project manager, Caroline Hurren, as well as Rhiannon Barker and Michael Cranna.

The MORI Health Research team was led by Kai Rudat and comprised Claire Ivins, Rezina Chowdhury and Lee Chan. Statistical support and advice was provided by Professor Roy Carr-Hill from the University of York.

The HEA would like to thank everyone who responded to the survey.

Introduction

The Chief Medical Officer's report for 1991 (Department of Health, 1992a) highlighted the health needs of black and minority ethnic groups. The report drew attention to considerable variations in disease patterns within and between ethnic groups. The need to provide appropriate services for these communities was emphasised, though it was acknowledged that the relevant information which would be needed to develop such services was, indeed, sparse. Publication in 1992 of the Government's white paper *The Health of the Nation* (Department of Health, 1992b) set a national strategy for health, including consideration of the particular needs of black and minority ethnic groups. Targets were set in five key areas: coronary heart disease and stroke, cancers, mental illness, HIV/AIDS and sexual health, and accidents. This was followed in 1993 with the publication of *Ethnicity and Health* (Balarajan and Raleigh, 1993) which highlighted the fact that these groups are at greater risk for most of the key areas identified in *The Health of the Nation*.

The Health Education Authority (HEA) aims to ensure that the people of England are more knowledgeable, better motivated and more able to acquire and maintain good health. As such, the HEA has a key role to play in the development of black and minority ethnic health issues.

However, whilst it had been involved for a number of years in the production of health education resources for black and minority ethnic groups, the HEA was also acutely aware that the needs of these communities had not been systematically assessed. In response to this, it began a multi-disciplinary programme of work to try to provide a positive basis for the development of black and minority ethnic group health issues. The programme of work had three main themes: alliance development activity, information services and research.

In 1993/94 the HEA ran a number of workshops for the NHS and other agencies to identify issues involved in meeting Health of the Nation targets for black and minority ethnic groups, and to develop health promotion strategies and opportunities for interventions. In September 1994 the HEA launched its database of health-related resources for black and minority ethnic groups and published the database in book form (Health Education Authority, 1994a).

Between 1992 and 1994 the HEA invested in a major programme of research to assess the knowledge, attitudes, behaviours and health status of the population in England. As part of the continuing commitment to black and minority ethnic groups it was decided to commit a substantial proportion of this investment specifically to research among some of the dominant ethnic communities in England. It is the results from the first wave of these studies which form the basis of this book.

Two health and lifestyles surveys were targeted at the general population, results of which are reported elsewhere (Health Education Authority, 1994b). These surveys show that, in the main, people in England are well informed about the health risks associated with practices such as smoking and engaging in unsafe sexual behaviours. The surveys also indicate that people are motivated to change the unhealthy aspects of their lifestyle. In this sense, the findings are encouraging. The results add to what is already known about the general population. However, such information has not to date been available for black and minority ethnic groups.

Most research on black and minority ethnic groups has tended to be disease-led, at the expense of a more encompassing perspective which would also integrate health beliefs, attitudes and behaviours. Studies show that there are some differences between black and minority ethnic groups and the population at large. South Asians, for instance, are more likely to die of coronary heart disease than the general population, whilst mortality rates from stroke are greater amongst people from the Caribbean, South Asia and the African Commonwealth (Balarajan and Raleigh, 1993). However, such studies fail to relate health status to situational and behavioural causes. Moreover, the majority of studies concentrate on one particular ethnic group, which makes comparison difficult.

It was to overcome some of these limitations that the HEA commissioned health and lifestyles surveys specifically for the black and minority ethnic groups. The black and minority ethnic groups' health and lifestyles survey reported here is the first national survey of knowledge, attitude, behaviour and health status of the black and minority ethnic groups in England. Five of the largest ethnic groups were targeted: African-Caribbeans, Bangladeshis, Indians/East African Asians, Pakistanis and Black Africans. The survey was based on extensive exploratory research (see Chapter 1), took into consideration the needs of the communities elucidated through focus groups and discussions with ethnic groups' representatives and experts, and made use of questionnaires which were administered in the community language of the respondents by bilingual interviewers. This survey provides the most complete and up-to-date comparative data on these ethnic groups and is a unique and extremely valuable source of information.

For comparative purposes, the HEA had planned to run the health and lifestyles survey targeting the general population and the black and minority ethnic groups in parallel and, as far as possible, address comparable issues – ideally using similar questions. However, there are limits to the comparisons which can be made between black and ethnic minority groups and the general population. Developmental work which preceded the survey suggested that some themes or questions used for the general population were either inappropriate or irrelevant for the black and minority ethnic groups targeted. Some sections of the survey, concerning topics such as language spoken, were central for many black and minority ethnic groups but unnecessary for the general population. However, as far as possible, the topic areas covered in the survey were identical to those used for the general population.

A wealth of information exists in the health and lifestyles survey. This report presents only the initial findings. More detailed analysis is being carried out and will be reported at a later date. In addition, the data from the survey will be made available at the ESRC data archive. The results of the second national black and minority ethnic group health and lifestyles survey, completed in late 1994 with a focus on nutrition and physical activity, will be reported in 1995.

The HEA has a major commitment to improving the health and well-being of the people of England. This report is the first to provide information on health-related knowledge, attitudes and behaviours of the black and minority ethnic groups in England. We hope it will prove to be a valuable source of information for NHS purchasers and providers in planning health promotion activities with black and minority ethnic groups; for local authorities and voluntary organisations working with different black and minority ethnic groups and for researchers interested in the health of minority ethnic groups. It will also provide a useful frame of reference for health-related data on minority ethnic groups collected at local level.

1. Background and methodology

Background

In August 1991 the Health Education Authority commissioned MORI's Health Research Unit to carry out a programme of health and lifestyle research on its behalf. The programme was intended to consist of separate quantitative surveys among the general public in the UK and among black and minority ethnic communities resident in the UK. The primary objective of the programme was to evaluate the HEA's key mission statement, that 'the people of England are more knowledgeable, better motivated and more able to acquire and maintain good health', by examining factors contributing to health status and assessing the needs, and the barriers to maintaining good health, of specific target groups. The research findings would inform the HEA's strategies for achieving Health of the Nation targets and for identifying and monitoring indicators as well as providing a frame of reference for data collected at local level.

The communities selected for inclusion in the first quantitative survey were African-Caribbeans, Black Africans, Indians and East African Asians, Pakistanis and Bangladeshis who make up the largest minority ethnic populations in England.

Given the need to obtain meaningful data for health education purposes, it was felt to be essential to carry out exploratory qualitative research in advance of the quantitative study.

Stages of the project

The study as a whole fell into a number of distinct stages:

- consultation with local community, academic and other experts
- qualitative research – group discussions and in-depth interviews
- developing a first draft of the questionnaire for the quantitative survey
- translating the questionnaire into the appropriate languages
- piloting all the different language versions of the questionnaire
- revising the questionnaires in the light of the pilot study
- main fieldwork
- data analysis.

Definition of terms

In this report we have used the term *African-Caribbean* to describe people who were born in or who have recent family origin in the West Indies and who have more distant family origins in Africa. (It does not include people of European or Asian origin whose families have been resident in the West Indies, nor does it include people with recent family origins in Africa.) By *Black African* we mean people with recent family origins in Africa – primarily those from both East and West African countries which are members of the New Commonwealth – and it excludes both people with family origins in North African countries and people of European or Asian family origin whose families have been resident in Africa. When we talk about *Indians*, *Pakistanis* or *Bangladeshis* we are referring to people who were born in or who have family origins in those countries; for this reason we sometimes use the term *Indians* to include those whose families were recently resident in African countries, though of Indian origin. By *East African Asians* we mean people of Indian family origin who were born in or whose families have recently resided in East African countries such as Uganda, Kenya and Tanzania.

Community consultation

A wide range of local community organisations and individuals were consulted over the research design. They included:

- 20 officers in 14 different local authorities, in roles such as community relations/ community services, equal opportunities, information and research

- 12 health and/or race-related organisations, such as Bradford Action on Health, Birmingham Health Promotion Unit, Linkworkers Association, King's Fund, and the Centre for Research on Ethnic Relations at Warwick University

- 11 voluntary organisations, such as the Asian Women's Forum, Confederation of Indian Organisations, local authorities' Race Relations Information Exchange.

The purpose of the consultation was to discuss the broad content of the study, especially topics which might prove sensitive; to get an initial feel for the health concerns of the various communities.

The qualitative research

The objectives of the qualitative research were:

- to establish the health issues of importance to black and minority ethnic communities, that is, including everyday health problems rather than focusing exclusively on major illnesses and diseases

- to examine awareness and experiences of, and attitudes towards, health-related services

- to determine the expectations of black and ethnic minority communities in their dealings with health and community services, and the extent to which these are met

- to establish attitudes to particular health and lifestyle issues:

    smoking
    ' alcohol
    sexual behaviour
    exercise and fitness
    diet and nutrition
    stress and psycho-social health

- to determine any barriers to achieving and maintaining a 'healthy' lifestyle which may exist in terms of:

    culture
    lifestyle
    religion
    language
    perceptions of health and disease

- to identify the main areas of health education needs within specific communities.

The research design was intended to take into account a complex mix of cultural, ethnic, class and life-stage factors. It was decided to use a needs-focused approach to the qualitative research, designed to provide in-depth coverage of those sectors within the communities which were clearly recognised as having the greatest needs and which were of particular relevance to the study (e.g. young people, mothers and so on).

Structure of the qualitative research

In total, twenty group discussions were carried out – fourteen with Asian groups, six with African-Caribbean groups – and twenty-two depth interviews with Black Africans, in the autumn and winter of 1991. Because of the greater heterogeneity of Black Africans, depth interviews, rather than focus groups, were chosen. The locations for this phase of the research were:

Pakistanis:	Bradford, Leicester
Bangladeshis:	Tower Hamlets
Indian Sikhs:	Southall, Leicester
East African Asians:	Harrow, Leicester
African-Caribbeans:	Birmingham, Brixton, Deptford
Black Africans:	Brixton, Stockwell, Peckham.

A number of the group discussions were conducted in the relevant Asian languages. All the moderators of the group discussions – some of whom were MORI researchers, while others were bilingual community contacts – were trained by MORI in qualitative research techniques, and matched to the groups in terms of gender and language. The locations and venues, together with the choice of language for the discussion, were chosen to replicate community patterns. The group discussions were structured by life-stage and social status, as well as by ethnic group; the depth interviews with Black Africans were structured by life-stage.

Qualitative research results

Results from the qualitative research were, as expected, complex in terms of the divergences in knowledge, attitude and behaviour displayed, both within and between each of the ethnic groups. Although, up to a point, a number of broad themes could be highlighted, it was clear that tailoring an appropriate standard set of questions to such a widely divergent audience would be a task fraught with difficulties.

Looking at the similarities, a number of broad themes emerged:

- respondents tended to view health holistically; their definition appeared to encompass concepts of mental and spiritual well-being. Worries and anxieties were cited by many as being a cause of ill health, although factors contributing to this varied between first and second generation UK residents. For the first generation at the top of their list of 'stressful' factors were financial stability, housing, employment, children's future, loss of cultural values, isolation and racism. For the second generation key factors were again employment and racism, but cultural conflict and education were also paramount.

- In terms of health services, misunderstandings and poor communication between GP and clients led to feelings of resignation, fatalism, the lowering of expectations and, on occasion, the exaggeration of symptoms. Respondents feared racial pigeon-holing, being treated as unintelligent or time-wasting. There was a consensus that a broader outlook from health professionals may help encompass some of the specific needs and priorities of black and minority ethnic groups.

- Although health considerations appeared to have limited influence on smoking, alcohol consumption and sexual behaviour, the main influences appeared to be cultural and social.

- Some areas of health-related behaviours carry cultural taboos for certain groups. The Sikh religion for example prohibits smoking, whilst Muslims do not allow alcohol consumption. In addition, for first generation Muslims and Sikhs the topic of sexual health was largely a taboo subject which would clearly be difficult to raise in an interview context.

Questionnaire development

Adapting the questionnaire in the light of qualitative research

The qualitative results presented challenges for those involved in the planning of the final questionnaire. The major dilemma when considering the format of the questionnaire was to find a balance between acknowledging 'community' priorities, as identified in the qualitative research, whilst at the same time maintaining a degree of comparability with questions which had been asked of the general population in the UK-wide Health and Lifestyles Survey (HEA, 1994b). From the point of view of obtaining data which could be used for prioritising public health services it was felt to be essential that data from ethnic minorities should be directly comparable to those collected from the general population. We hope that we were able to strike the balance.

In relation to health services, access to services was acknowledged as a key area. A considerable amount of time was allocated to the health services section, with questions included on ease of and language of communication with health professionals, provision of interpreters, assessment of treatment and use of alternative healers. Given reportedly high rates of illiteracy in certain groups questions on literacy were added.

Consideration of questions on health-related behaviours proved more problematic. Although it was acknowledged that it may be offensive, for example, to ask Sikhs about smoking behaviour, it was realised that there may be discrepancies between culturally-held values and personal behaviours (particularly amongst the younger generation). It was decided therefore to retain questions on smoking so that comparisons could be made with general population data. Interviewers were briefed that sensitivity may be needed when covering these topics. In the case of smoking, to make specific questions more appropriate, consideration was given as to whether to include questions on the chewing of tobacco-related products.

To accommodate the additional questions that were added, other questions felt to be of a lower priority, which had been asked of the general population, were excluded from this particular survey.

Considerable debate focused on the section on sexual health. It was clear from the qualitative work that sexual health would be particularly sensitive to the older generation of Muslims and Sikhs. There were strong feelings that the survey should not result in offence being given to the communities being researched. Yet, there was a recognition that unless we attempted to ask certain questions we would firstly never have a real feeling for the force of resistance to certain issues being raised, and more importantly we would lose valuable data on knowledge, attitudes and behaviours concerning sexual health, on which to base future educational campaigns. Fuelled both by the argument that purported fear of creating further stigma has led to a degree of paralysis among health educators in tackling issues surrounding sexual health for people from black and minority ethnic communities, together with the importance of being able to compare data with the general population, a decision was made to pilot the same questions on sexual health as had been asked of the general population.

A particularly difficult issue to grapple with in relation to sexual health (which also applies though maybe to a lesser extent in other areas) is that of generational differences. It was evident that a number of questions which would be answered by the younger generation would be refused by older people. In terms of sexual health, looking at risk groups for diseases and unwanted pregnancies, the key target group for health educators is the 16 to 25 year age group. It was assumed that this group would be more ready to answer questions perceived as offensive by their elders. When debating whether or not to modify questions for the survey it has to be acknowledged that the resulting questionnaire is always a compromise.

The draft questionnaire consisted of a number of modules:

- demographic information (about the respondent and his/her household)
- communications

- self-reported health status

- health concerns

- home and local environment

- psycho-social health and social support

- awareness, use and experiences of GP services

- health promotion issues

- self-reported health information needs

- cancer screening

- smoking.

In a separate self-completion questionnaire, knowledge, behaviour and attitudes on sexual health issues were covered.

Translation

Given that a significant number of people from the black and minority ethnic communities either do not speak, or are not comfortable with speaking, English, the questionnaire had to be translated. One of the major difficulties encountered was which language to translate into.

It was felt important to take on board the experiences of other researchers who had done survey work requiring translations into Asian languages. The experiences of the Linguistic Minorities Project in the Adult Language Use Survey, as reported in *The Other Languages of England* (Stubbs, 1985), were particularly valuable.

Asian languages

A wide range of different languages are spoken by people of Indian and East African Asian origin living in this country; this is true to a lesser extent of people of Pakistani origin. Some of the main Asian languages spoken in the UK do not have a written form, practically speaking. We therefore had to make difficult decisions about how many languages and which ones the survey fieldwork should be carried out in, given that we could not accommodate all the possible language requirements. We wanted to interview people in the languages they spoke at home – the languages which they were most at their ease communicating in, and which would interpose the least barrier between interviewer and respondent. This meant using regional rather than national languages wherever possible.

The languages of most relevance for Indians and East African Asians are Gujerati and Punjabi written in the Gurmukhi script, often referred to as Punjabi (G). Most Bangladeshis in this country speak Sylheti, a regional variant of Bengali, but one which does not have a written form of its own; the language of literacy is Bengali. We therefore had to use Bengali as the written medium but with the terms closest to those which would be used by Sylheti-speakers wherever possible. The Bengali version of the questionnaire would also be used with Indians who were native Bengali speakers (for example those originating from the Indian state of West Bengal).

Like the researchers of the Linguistic Minorities Project (LMP), the MORI researchers experienced their greatest difficulties in finding the best language in which to interview people of Pakistani origin. The mother tongue of most Pakistanis in the UK is Punjabi, often referred to in this context as Punjabi (Urdu) or Punjabi (U). It is not true to say that Punjabi (U) does not have a written form, but for most practical purposes, including survey work, it might as well not have one. Punjabi (U) *can* be written (in the Perso-Arabic script, like Urdu) but is rarely written in the Pakistani Punjab and almost never in the UK; the language of literacy is Urdu. However, some Pakistani men and many Pakistani women are not fluent speakers, let alone readers, of Urdu.

The LMP researchers found that many of their Punjabi-speaking interviewers, especially the younger ones, had limited reading skills in Punjabi, and as a result they opted for a questionnaire in Punjabi written in the Perso-Arabic script but supplemented this with a Punjabi questionnaire transliterated into English and an audio-cassette of someone reading the Punjabi text aloud. The MORI research team at first opted for a similar approach and indeed got as far as having the questionnaire for the pilot study translated into Punjabi in the Perso-Arabic script. However, MORI needed large numbers of interviewers with at least some reading skills in Punjabi (U) if it was going to be a viable option as a written language, because of the large scale of the project. The difficulties in recruiting sufficient numbers of interviewers with such skills – eleven or twelve years after the Adult Language Use Survey – proved insurmountable. (Many people tried to tell us that there was 'no such thing' as written Punjabi (U).) We also came across considerable resistance to the idea of using Punjabi (U) in an 'official' way, and especially to the idea of using it as the primary means of interviewing Pakistanis, because of the perceived higher status of Urdu. We therefore had to accept that all the written survey instruments were going to have to be in Urdu, and that our interviewers would have to supplement the Urdu version with Punjabi as required.

Our final choice of Asian languages was therefore Gujerati, Punjabi (G), Bengali and Urdu (backed up orally by Punjabi).

The translations were carried out by an agency specialising in Asian languages, and back-checked by community consultants who were part of the MORI research team. It was agreed that the style used in the translations should be simple, clear and straightforward, and that the language used should be as similar as possible to that used in everyday speech in Britain, and accessible to those with little formal education.

Black Africans

Black Africans living in the UK are an extremely heterogeneous group, with origins in a large number of different countries. Across this group a large number of different languages are spoken: for example, among Nigerians alone, we would find speakers of Yoruba, Twi and Ibo, and others. However, English is widely spoken as a lingua franca by many people of African origin living in Britain. We therefore concluded that it would be reasonable to attempt to interview all our Black African respondents in English.

African-Caribbeans

Although English is not the only language spoken by people of African-Caribbean origin – members of the older generation in particular may speak French, French-based creole/patwa or English-based creole – on the available evidence it seemed reasonable to assume that the vast majority of African-Caribbeans would be fluent speakers of English.

Piloting

The questionnaires (main questionnaire and self-completion) were piloted in a number of different locations among all the target ethnic groups for the survey, in July and August 1992. For the pilot study, sampling points were drawn in areas where the 1981 Census indicated a fairly high concentration of the target ethnic minority groups. Interviewers were asked to screen addresses in these points in order to find suitable respondents. The Gujerati version was piloted in the Wembley area, north-west London; the Bengali version in Tower Hamlets, East London; the Punjabi (G) and Urdu versions in Bradford; the English version was piloted among Asian respondents in all these locations and was also piloted among African-Caribbean and Black African respondents in Lambeth, south-west London. For the Asian target groups, native speakers of the relevant languages were paired with English-speaking interviewers in order to carry out both the screening and the interviewing; each pair of interviewers was asked to carry out interviews both in English and in the relevant Asian language, and to encourage Asian respondents to be interviewed in their mother tongue, if necessary, in order to make sure that survey materials were well tested in all languages. The interviewers were briefed and debriefed in person in London and Bradford.

The pilot study was invaluable not only in obtaining reactions to the particular questions used but also for general experience of interviewing respondents from traditional Asian backgrounds who speak little or no English. A questionnaire which typically took around sixty minutes among native English speakers in many cases took two hours, or even longer, among the respondents for the pilot study, and we felt it was important to look at the reasons for this.

- Many respondents had no idea what population surveys or social research was, and most had not heard of MORI nor of the HEA. Interviewers had to provide far more introductory information for respondents – about themselves and the organisation they worked for, what the HEA was and the purpose of the survey, countering suggestions that they were from the DSS, the council, to do with poll tax, etc. – than they would expect to do in the course of their usual survey work, and this was a time-consuming process. As a result of this we felt there was a need for an information sheet for respondents, explaining in a simple question-and-answer format some basic facts about survey research and giving reassurance about confidentiality.

- Traditions of hospitality meant that respondents often kindly offered the interviewers tea and other refreshments, and while the interviewers appreciated both the refreshments and the kind intentions, this did prolong the interviewing process.

- When terms were used which people did not understand, either in English or in one of the other survey languages, they often wanted the interviewer to explain what the term meant and give some information about it – examples of this would be 'well-woman clinic' and 'cervical smear test'. The interviewer therefore had to be prepared either to give an explanation (interviewers are trained not to give any 'unauthorised' information to assist a respondent in answering a question) or to spend time explaining why they could not give an explanation – without, of course, giving offence.

- In some communities we found few respondents were able to read showcards (visual prompts) either in English or in their mother tongue. Where this happened, the interviewer had to read out each item on the showcard to the respondent and obtain a 'yes/no' answer on each. Showcards are very widely used in survey research in the UK in the expectation that virtually all respondents will be able to deal confidently with them and that they will provide an efficient way of getting a lot of questions answered in a short space of time. However, for respondents who are not fluent readers, showcards can be intimidating and tiring, and therefore counterproductive.

As well as the length of the interview and the reasons for this, some other valuable points emerged:

- A wide range of terms were not generally understood in some communities: these included 'stress', 'lack of personal space', 'environmental pollution', 'healthy foods', and many medical terms such as 'diabetes', 'gangrene', 'degenerative illness'. We found that in some cases it was the concepts which were untranslatable, and that where respondents were familiar with the concepts, they tended to use the English words for them.

- Some standard survey research terms and concepts such as 'household' and 'head of household' proved difficult to use in the standard way, because of the very flexible composition of some Asian households, and also because interviewers came across not only 'extended families' but also 'extended addresses' consisting of a number of houses side-by-side in which some of these extended families lived.

- When trying to elicit information about household income, benefits received by the household, or the occupation of the head of the household, difficulties with the definition of 'household' became particularly acute. The interviewers also found that respondents who were not the head of the household themselves were unlikely to know the answers to these questions.

- It was impossible to get a private interview with the respondent in some households, especially where there were large families. Interviewers found themselves having to ask questions on potentially sensitive or embarrassing issues when members of the respondent's family were present in the same room. Family members often wanted to become involved in the interview – husbands wanting to respond on behalf of wives, and vice versa, and also parents on behalf of children. The interviewers reported that some Asian women respondents, especially older ones, would not answer questions on gynaecological matters, and the circumstances were not conducive to any discussion of problems with relationships or family members.

- Given the cultural and religious strictures in some of the Asian communities on some of the behaviours and issues addressed in the questionnaire, and the lack of privacy during the interview, it was not surprising that many respondents were reluctant to discuss topics such as smoking. The self-completion questionnaire on sexual health met with very little success among the Asian communities – there were significant problems both with respondents being unable to read the questionnaire, and with those who could read it having strong objections to its coverage. The self-completion questionnaire was most acceptable to young people, those educated in the UK and with good literacy skills in English. The pilot interviewers reported that in one tight-knit community, word spread rapidly about the content of the self-completion questionnaire after they had spent one day interviewing there, so that on subsequent days they found a much higher rate of refusals to take part in the survey.

Questionnaire revision

Following the pilot study, two slightly different versions of the main questionnaire were developed. One was the version intended for use with Black African and African-Caribbean respondents, where question wordings were kept comparable with those used in the general public survey. The other was the version for use with respondents from the Asian communities, and was much shorter than the general public questionnaire, with some questions amended to exclude terms which had caused particular difficulty at the pilot stage.

Similarly, the version of the self-completion questionnaire intended for use with Black Africans and African-Caribbeans remained identical to that used in the general public survey, while the one for Asian respondents was both shortened and significantly changed, in an effort to make it more widely acceptable, for example by placing questions about knowledge and attitudes on sexual health issues before the questions about behaviour.

Fieldwork documents

Two monolingual versions of the main questionnaire were produced – one for African-Caribbeans and Black Africans, the other for Asian respondents who had English as their main spoken language or preferred to be interviewed in English. Four bilingual versions of the 'Asian' questionnaire were also produced, each of which had the translated text calligraphed on to a version of the questionnaire which also gave all the question wordings in English (we knew that some respondents would want to switch languages depending on the subjects they were discussing). Similarly, four monolingual versions of the self-completion questionnaire were produced – one each for African-Caribbean/African men, African-Caribbean/African women, Asian men, Asian women – together with eight bilingual versions where translated text was typeset on to the questionnaires together with the text in English. We produced sets of showcards for each of the survey languages, and these were all typeset, to ensure that they were clearly legible to both interviewers and respondents.

Main fieldwork

Sampling strategy

Our aim was find a sampling strategy which would enable the survey to cover the majority of people belonging to the target ethnic groups and to achieve large numbers of interviews in each, without stretching the fieldwork budget to an unacceptable extent. We were significantly hampered by the fact that data from the 1991 Census were not available during the period in which the sample had to be drawn. We had to rely on 1981 Census information, where the best proxy we could find for data on ethnicity was information on the country of birth of heads of household. Furthermore, we anticipated that there would be difficulties with the definition of some of the ethnic groups of interest to us. For example, we were unable to draw a clear distinction between people of Indian and African family origin born in East Africa; nor could we distinguish between people of European and African family origin born in other African countries of the New Commonwealth.

Information from the 1981 Census was used to identify a universe of Census enumeration districts (EDs) where 10% or more of the ED's population lived in households where the head of household was born in

- the West Indies or Guyana

- India

- Pakistan

- Bangladesh

- East Africa (New Commonwealth)

- other African countries belonging to the New Commonwealth.

Five interlocking samples were then drawn from this universe (one for each of the target ethnic groups). For sampling purposes, we assumed that the majority of those with heads of household born in East Africa would be people of Indian family origin, so the samples for Indians and East Africans were combined. The sample for each target group consisted of EDs where at least 10% of the population lived in households headed by a member of that ethnic group, with varying penetrations of other target ethnic groups. The number of EDs in each group's sample was in line with the number of interviews we were aiming to achieve: 800 with African-Caribbeans, 400 with Black Africans, 1000 Indians and East African Asians, 800 Pakistanis and 500 Bangladeshis.

The overall sample consisted of 354 EDs, with 65 addresses from the Small Users' Postcode Address File selected at random within each ED. Only one sample point fell outside England.

Data from the 1991 Census subsequently confirmed that choosing EDs with a minimum penetration of 10% of residents from these minority ethnic groups does indeed give access to the majority of people belonging to these minority ethnic groups who are resident in urban areas. If we take urban to mean London, other metropolitan areas plus district councils which are defined as cities (such as Leicester), we find that 85% of African-Caribbeans, 79% of Indians, 75% of Pakistanis and 82% of Bangladeshis resident in England live in urban areas of this kind. In addition, we included in our definition of 'urban' other towns with significant black and minority ethnic populations (such as some Lancashire mill towns). The revised universe covers 88% of African-Caribbeans, 86% of Indians, 88% of Pakistanis, and 88% of Bangladeshis.

The proportion of African-Caribbeans resident in such urban areas who live in EDs with a minimum penetration of 10% is 74%; the corresponding figures for Indians, Pakistanis and Bangladeshis are 78%, 86% and 85% respectively.

The fieldforce

MORI's national fieldforce provided all fieldwork services for the quantitative survey. For this survey, we needed interviewers with a great deal of experience of random, preselected survey methodologies who would be able to carry out most of the screening of addresses and some of the interviewing. We also needed interviewers who had good literacy skills both in English and one of the other survey languages, as well as being fluent speakers of both, to assist with the screening where necessary, and to carry out the interviewing in Asian languages. Over the spring and summer of 1992 we therefore recruited and trained about a hundred new interviewers with bilingual skills. Many of the interviewers who worked on this project had already worked on the parallel survey among the general population. All interviewers were given full personal briefings on all aspects of the survey by members of the MORI research team at a series of regional meetings, as well as written instructions and background notes.

Screening and interviewing

All sample addresses were screened by MORI interviewers. Those which were identifiable as invalid (non-residential, vacant, demolished, etc.) were eliminated from the sample. Addresses were screened for multiple households, and if necessary a random selection grid (Kish grid) was used to select one of the households resident at the address.

Selected households were then screened for ethnicity – this process is described in more detail below. Where households contained people from one or more of the target ethnic groups for the survey, the interviewer then went on to obtain a listing of all adults eligible to take part in the survey (i.e. household members aged between 16 and 74, normally resident at the address, and belonging to one or other of the target ethnic groups). Households containing only people aged 75+ were eliminated at this stage. In households where there was more than one potential respondent, the intended respondent was then selected using a Kish grid.

Where necessary, bilingual interviewers completed the household screening, and potential respondents were offered the option of being interviewed in any one of the survey languages. Respondents were also offered a gender-matched interviewer where this was appropriate.

After completing the face-to-face interview, respondents in the 16 to 54 age range and who had said they could read at least one of the survey languages were handed a self-completion questionnaire, together with an envelope. They were asked by the interviewer to fill in the questionnaire on their own, put it into the envelope and seal it before handing the envelope back to the interviewer. Interviewers did not look at the completed questionnaire at any stage, and therefore could not tell to what extent the respondent had actually filled it in.

The respondent's unique identifying number was written on the envelope. At the office, the identifying number was transferred to the questionnaire itself and some basic editing was carried out. It was at this stage that questionnaires which were mostly blank were identified. Self-completion questionnaires were then sent for data entry and matched back to the main questionnaire with which they belonged, via the unique identifying number.

Screening for ethnicity

This was one of the most difficult and sensitive parts of the interviewers' work; we had to try to ensure that we used terms which were acceptable, easily understood and meaningful. Interviewers showed informants a showcard where the following descriptions were listed:

> Caribbean/West Indian
> Black African
> Indian
> Pakistani
> Bangladeshi
> East African Asian.

They asked the informant whether anyone in his or her household was from any of the ethnic groups on the card, and if they received an answer in the affirmative they continued the screening by enumerating all the people in the household who were aged 16–74 inclusive and who belonged to any one of those groups. If the informant responded by describing people in the household as Kenyan Asians, Ugandan Asians or something similar, interviewers were told that they could code this response as East African Asian. If the informant did not give an affirmative answer to any of the categories shown but said that there were people in the household who were Black British, British Asian or of mixed race/parentage, then the interviewers were instructed to probe further by asking if either of the parents of the people concerned was from one of the ethnic groups listed; if they received an affirmative answer to this question, then the interviewer coded the relevant parental origin and proceeded to enumerate the household members eligible to participate in the survey.

Interviewers were trained only to list and select respondents from those people in the household who were eligible to participate in the survey both on the grounds of their ethnic origin and their age. Individuals living in households where there was someone belonging to one of the target ethnic groups for the survey but who were not themselves members of one of these groups were not listed in the household enumeration; neither were individuals who belonged to one of the target ethnic groups but who were under 16 or over 74 years of age.

One slight complication was that (as anticipated from the experiences of other researchers) the interviewers found that some older people from the Asian communities did not know their exact ages – their date of birth had never been recorded. In these circumstances, the interviewer accepted the estimate of the person concerned or of a close relative.

Response rates

In total, 23 022 addresses were issued, of which 4477 (19%) turned out to be voids (non-residential, boarded up, etc.). At the addresses which were not voids, 1427 people refused to give any information about their household, and at 2580 the interviewer was unable to make contact with any adult resident despite four or more calls (8% and 14% respectively of non-void addresses). In 9543 cases the screened households were definitely identified as not containing any eligible respondents for the survey (51% of non-void addresses); 53 of these contained only members of the ethnic groups of interest who were aged 75+ and therefore ineligible by age.

The screening process identified 4571 addresses containing an eligible potential respondent. Among the potential respondents, 501 refused to be interviewed (11%), 384 could not be contacted in person by the interviewer despite repeated calls (8%), and 137 could not be interviewed for other reasons, such as being ill or away during the fieldwork period in each area or needing to be interviewed in a language other than English, Punjabi, Urdu, Gujerati or Bengali/Sylheti. Interviews were carried out with 3549 respondents (i.e. at 78% of valid screened addresses), though 31 of these interviews were later rejected because the data were not sufficiently complete. The screening process is summarised in the table, and outcomes broken down by the ethnic group of households. The summary also shows the proportion of interviews conducted in the mother tongue (Indians – 32%; Pakistanis – 50%; Bangladeshis – 70%).

The screening process

		%
Total number of addresses issued	23 022	100
Voids (non-residential, vacant)	4 477	19
Non-voids	18 545	100
Refused to give any information about household	1 427	8
Unable to make contact with any adult resident after 4+ calls	2 580	14
Addresses definitely not containing members of any target group	9 490	51
Other failures	360	2
Addresses definitely containing members of target groups	4 688	

Response rate by ethnic group of leads identified

	African- Caribbeans	Black Africans	Indians/ EAA	Pakistanis	Bangladeshis
Identified	1 084	293	1363	1196	752
– 75+ only	14	1	11	3	1
– ill/away	15	9	28	19	16
Valids	1 055	283	1324	1174	735
– refusals	164	38	173	94	32
– non-contacts	152	37	106	60	29
Successful interviews	729	202	1 017	935	667
Successful as % of screened, eligible respondents	69	71	77	80	91
Proportion of interviews conducted in mother tongue	NA	NA	32	50	70

The response rate to the self-completion questionnaire was significantly lower than that to the main questionnaire, with a higher proportion of outright refusals among all the ethnic groups covered by the survey but particularly among the three Asian communities, as might have been anticipated. There were also a substantial number of respondents unable to read either English or their mother tongue sufficiently well to be able to complete it; again, it was anticipated that this would be the case, but in the event the number of people describing themselves as unable to read the questionnaire was higher than would have been expected from responses to direct questions about languages spoken, read and written. In the survey carried out among the general population, around 95% of survey respondents in the 16 to 54 age range agreed to fill in the self-completion questionnaire.

Response rate to self-completion questionnaire

	African- Caribbeans	Black Africans	Indians/ EAA	Pakistanis	Bangladeshis
Total eligible by age	499	185	839	812	568
	%	%	%	%	%
Refused	18	17	33	26	34
Unable to read questionnaire	1	8	10	30	25
Accepted	77	74	56	43	36

Survey data

Survey data have been edited and then weighted in two different ways:

- by household size – each respondent received a weight proportional to the number of adults aged 16–74 in their household, to correct for the fact that MORI only interviewed one adult per household, thereby lessening the chances of selection for adults in larger households

- by age within gender within region (Greater London versus the rest of Great Britain), using 1991 Census data to calculate target weights.

The tabulations have been formatted to exclude people for whom there was no answer recorded for a particular question from the base for that question when calculating percentage findings.

The findings contained in this report cover the key sections of the questionnaire (demographics, communications, health status, use of services, and smoking behaviour). Other data will be presented in separate publications.

The analysis in this report focuses on comparisons between the different black and minority ethnic communities, and with the UK-wide Health and Lifestyles Survey. Because of the small sample size of Black Africans, this group was excluded from the analysis. Further comparisons are shown for age and gender. Other variables, such as languages spoken, educational status, etc. will be analysed and reported separately.

Many surveys ask questions about race and ethnicity of people. This has caused concern among members of some ethnic communities about the way in which data collected on race and ethnicity may be used to stereotype black and minority ethnic people. These concerns are acknowledged by the HEA. The purpose of the present survey is not to highlight differences but to look into certain forms of interdependence and coherence in behaviours, attitudes and norms – in short, lifestyles – and their relation to health. It is only in so far as lifestyles are expected to vary according to ethnicity that it is appropriate to select this variable to describe very complex forms of social differentiation. The data collected have been systematically compared to those on the general population in order to identify differences which can serve as the basis for interventions better tailored to the needs of all people.

Statistical significance

As with all sample surveys, the results are subject to sampling tolerances. Because of the complexity of the sample design, and the relatively small size of each target group sample, it has not been possible to estimate design effects.

For a pure random sample, the following sampling tolerances would apply:

	Confidence interval* for findings at or near these percentages		
	10% or 90% ±%	30% or 70% ±%	50% ±%
Indians (N = 1017)	1.8	2.8	3.1
Pakistanis (N = 935)	1.9	2.9	3.2
African-Caribbeans (N = 729)	2.2	3.3	3.6
Bangladeshis (N = 667)	2.3	3.5	3.8

*based on 95% confidence interval

A cautious adjustment for likely design effects would be to increase these tolerance intervals by a factor of 1.3.

2. Demographic factors

This chapter profiles our sample of the four target communities. It shows respondents' characteristics on the key demographic variables such as age and gender, work status, educational status, and housing status. The most important section of this chapter focuses on information about respondents' linguistic status. This includes self-assessments of the languages spoken by the target communities, as well as questions about literacy.

The demographic information contained in this section is not intended to provide new insights. Other data sources, such as the 1991 Census, have already profiled the characteristics of the different black and minority ethnic communities. Where appropriate, we have drawn comparisons with such information. These comparisons serve to confirm the representativeness of our sample, as well as highlight key differences between the national coverage of the Census, and the coverage of this survey, which has an urban focus (see Chapter 1).

Age and gender profile

Table 1 shows the number of successful interviews for each of the ethnic groups and their demographic sub-groups (see Table 1 unweighted section). The second part of the table shows the weighted population figures. OPCS Census figures for each of the black and minority ethnic target groups were used to construct the weight matrix. Comparisons of the unweighted and weighted figures show that significant weight factors had to be applied for men in the 16–29 year old age band. This group is commonly under-represented in social surveys, as a result of lower contact rates, high mobility, and higher refusal rates. Amongst male African-Caribbeans, there also was a significantly lower participation rate amongst those aged 30 to 49. With these exceptions, the survey coverage closely reflects Census profiles.

The achieved sample sizes for each of the ethnic community groups allow for meaningful comparisons both between the groups, and with known UK figures. Some of the individual sub-groups (especially Pakistani and Bangladeshi women aged 50 to 74 years) have very small bases. As a result some of the comparisons in this report will need to be treated with some caution. Only findings which are statistically significant are commented on in the text of the report.

Table 1: Unweighted and weighted age profile

	Unweighted				Weighted			
	African-Caribbean N	Indian N	Pakistani N	Bangladeshi N	African-Caribbean N	Indian N	Pakistani N	Bangladeshi N
Women	432	527	471	350	369	507	448	315
16–29	144	172	195	145	148	180	200	150
30–49	148	247	220	147	138	228	182	122
50–74	140	108	56	58	83	99	66	43
Men	276	490	456	315	340	511	480	350
16–29	76	144	157	105	130	170	191	145
30-49	70	219	202	118	111	228	184	102
50–74	130	127	97	92	99	113	105	103
Total	708	1 017	927	665	709	1 018	928	665

Country of birth

The age groups covered in this survey are 16 to 74 year olds. Table 2 shows the proportion of the three age bands used in the analysis, who were either born in the UK or outside the UK. For African-Caribbeans, there is almost an even split between those born in the UK (47%) and those born in the West Indies (53%). In the youngest age band, 86% were born in the UK; this falls to 33% of 30 to 49 year olds and to 1% of those aged 50 to 74 years. For the different South Asian communities, the proportions born in the UK are significantly lower (19% for Indians, 20% for Pakistanis, and 9% for Bangladeshis). For Indians and Pakistanis, approximately half of those aged 16 to 29 were born in the UK. Amongst Bangladeshis, one in five of this age group were born in the UK. Beyond age 29, almost all of the South Asians covered in this survey were born outside the UK.

23

Table 2: Country of birth (Source: AS Q13a; AC Q18)

Ethnic group	Country of birth	All %	16–29 %	30–49 %	50–74 %
African-Caribbean	West Indies/Guyana	53	11	66	97
	UK	47	86	33	1
	Other	<0.5	3	1	2
Indian	India	56	33	62	79
	UK	19	50	3	0
	East Africa	20	14	30	9
	Other	8	3	5	12
Pakistani	Pakistan	74	52	89	91
	UK	20	45	2	1
	Other	6	3	9	8
Bangladeshi	Bangladesh	91	81	98	99
	UK	9	19	1	0
	Other	<0.5	0	1	1

Base: All adults

Table 3 shows the Census data for place of birth for the four target communities. Our survey figures correspond closely with the data derived from the Census, even when allowing for the slightly different construction for the age bands used.

Table 3: Census analysis of place of birth (Source: OPCS)

Ethnic group	Place of birth	All %	Under 16 %	16–29 %	30–44 %	45–64 %	65 and over %
African-Caribbean	UK	54	97	91	29	5	9
	Outside UK	46	3	9	71	95	91
Indian	UK	42	95	52	5	2	5
	Outside UK	58	5	48	95	98	95
Pakistani	UK	51	88	48	5	3	7
	Outside UK	49	12	52	95	97	93
Bangladeshi	UK	37	67	18	4	3	9
	Outside UK	63	33	82	96	97	91

Languages spoken

Many service providers who have significant minority ethnic communities within their area of responsibility are concerned about communication strategies with the different minority ethnic communities. In the health sector there are a large number of initiatives aimed at minority ethnic communities in general, and at non-English speakers in particular. These include the production of written materials, the use of mother-tongue materials in audio or video format, and local community or service-based provision of link-workers, interpreters, and advocates. Whilst there is a strong awareness amongst service planners and providers of the need for mother-tongue or bilingual communication approaches, there is no reliable measure of need. There have been some small-scale assessments carried out by individual health authorities (for example the multi-lingual residents survey carried out by MORI's Health Research Unit in East London (CELFHSA/MORI, 1993)), but there has not been any large-scale assessment since the Linguistic Minorities Project in the early 1980s (Stubbs, 1985), and the 1982 Black and White Britain Survey (Brown, 1984). Both surveys highlighted the fact that significant proportions of black and minority ethnic communities spoke little or no English. For example, the Black and White Britain Survey shows that the proportion who speak little or no English is 76% amongst Bangladeshi women, 70% amongst Pakistani women, 50% amongst Bangladeshi men, and 42% amongst Indian women.

The current survey provides the first opportunity to update these figures. In addition, it collected more detailed information on other languages spoken, as well as literacy. It should be added, however, that all of the measures were respondents' self-assessments.

Table 4 shows the extent to which English and a number of the key mother-tongue languages are spoken by the three South Asian communities. Amongst Indians, 85% report to be able to speak English. Amongst Indian men, English is spoken almost universally (ranging from 96% of 16 to 29 year olds to 86% of those aged 50 to 74). Amongst Indian women, high proportions in the 16 to 29 year old age band (89%) and in the 30 to 49 year old age band (80%) report to be able to speak English. Only amongst women aged 50 to 74 do less than half (47%) report that they can speak English.

The key mother-tongue languages spoken amongst the Indian sub-group are Gujerati (50%) and Punjabi (43%). This reflects the two regional sub-groups contained within the Indian community which are Punjabi-speaking Sikhs, and Indians who have migrated from the Gujerat region either directly to the UK, or via East Africa. Smaller proportions report to be able to speak Hindi (33%) or Urdu (15%). The proportions who report to be able to speak the two regional languages (Gujerati and Punjabi) are consistent across men and women, and across the different age bands.

Amongst Pakistanis, identical proportions report to be able to speak Urdu (75%), Punjabi (73%), and English (72%). Reported English-speaking competence declines across age bands from 95% of young men to 66% of men aged 50 to 74; amongst women the decline is much more dramatic; from 78% to 15% respectively. Again, ability to speak Punjabi or Urdu is much more consistent across men and women and the different age bands.

Amongst the Bangladeshi community, the proportion who report to be able to speak English is significantly lower (59%). The most frequently mentioned language is Bengali (90%), and a further 24% mention Sylheti, with an additional 19% also reporting to be able to speak Urdu. Amongst Bangladeshi women, only amongst the youngest age group is English spoken by a majority (68%). Clearly, Bengali and/or Sylheti is the key language medium for this community.

Table 4: Languages spoken (Source: AS Q14)

Ethnic group	Language	All %	Women 16–29 %	Women 30–49 %	Women 50–74 %	Men 16–29 %	Men 30-49 %	Men 50–74 %
Indian	English	85	89	80	47	96	93	86
	Gujerati	50	45	54	49	46	54	49
	Punjabi	43	46	40	45	48	42	36
	Hindi	33	20	38	40	18	45	39
	Urdu	15	14	10	9	13	22	24
Pakistani	Punjabi	73	70	78	84	69	73	72
	English	72	78	42	15	95	94	66
	Urdu	75	74	72	68	69	84	80
Bangladeshi	Bengali	90	90	85	79	92	90	95
	English	59	68	21	10	92	72	51
	Sylheti	24	22	33	36	15	24	23
	Urdu	19	13	10	6	18	24	38

Base: All adults

Table 5 provides further information on which language respondents from the different communities perceive as their main language. The table shows the linguistic 'segmentation' of the different South Asian communities. Amongst Indians, around a third (32%) consider English to be their main spoken language. The remainder of this group divides into the two regional sub-groups of Gujeratis and Punjabi-speaking Sikhs. The linguistic segmentation is even more pronounced, when looking at age differences. For the younger group of Indians, English emerges as the main spoken language, whilst amongst the older age group, it is overtaken in importance by Gujerati and Punjabi.

A similar pattern of segmentation can be seen for the Pakistani community. Here, Punjabi is the single most significant language (mentioned by 48%). Certainly for those aged 30 or over, it is the main spoken language. English is mentioned by a quarter of Pakistanis, but it is only amongst the younger age groups, especially young men (58%) where it is more likely to be perceived as the main spoken language.

By contrast, the Bangladeshi community presents a much more homogeneous picture when it comes to the analysis of the main spoken language. In total, three-quarters (73%) identify Bengali as their main spoken language. There is very little variation by either gender or age in this stated preference. English is mentioned by one in ten as the main spoken language, with the highest preference identified by young men (25%).

Table 5: Main spoken language (Source: AS Q15)

		All	Women			Men		
			16–29	30–49	50–74	16–29	30-49	50–74
Ethnic group	Language	%	%	%	%	%	%	%
Indian	Gujerati	36	28	45	45	18	44	37
	English	32	51	18	8	62	25	19
	Punjabi	24	16	29	33	16	24	29
	Urdu	3	3	3	2	1	4	5
	Hindi	2	0	1	4	1	1	6
Pakistani	Punjabi	48	34	66	84	28	51	57
	English	24	37	3	0	58	15	7
	Urdu	22	23	26	16	10	27	30
Bangladeshi	Bengali	73	72	72	71	68	76	83
	Sylheti	17	14	27	28	7	17	17
	English	10	14	1	0	25	7	0

Base: All adults

Table 6 shows which language is spoken in respondents' homes. The figures very much mirror those described above, with the same age and gender differences amongst Indians and Pakistanis, and a more consistent pattern emerging for Bangladeshis.

Table 6: Language spoken at home (Source: AS Q16)

		All	Women			Men		
			16–29	30–49	50–74	16–29	30-49	50–74
Ethnic group	Language	%	%	%	%	%	%	%
Indian	Gujerati	44	39	47	45	40	48	46
	English	35	51	29	5	56	31	24
	Punjabi	34	37	35	34	34	32	31
	Urdu	4	3	3	3	2	5	4
	Hindi	3	1	3	8	2	2	3
Pakistani	Punjabi	60	51	63	84	54	60	62
	Urdu	34	41	33	26	28	33	39
	English	22	25	12	0	39	17	22
Bangladeshi	Bengali	80	81	69	69	86	81	83
	Sylheti	20	16	32	33	11	20	19
	English	8	14	4	0	15	6	1

Base: All adults

Languages read

For many service providers, written materials form an important plank of their communications strategies with service users. Tables 7–9 show which languages are read by the different South Asian communities, which languages people prefer to read, and their self-assessment of their literacy level in English.

Table 7 shows that amongst the Indian community, 76% report to be able to read English. Around a third (34%) report to be able to read Gujerati, and 21% report to be able to read Punjabi in the Gurmukhi script. Only 18% report that they read Hindi. Small proportions mention Urdu (8%), and Punjabi in the Urdu script (5%). A further 5% state that they cannot read any of the languages asked about. For Indian men English is clearly the most frequently mentioned language in which respondents are literate (ranging from 96% of younger men to 71% of those aged 50 to 74). For women, the decline of literacy in English is more pronounced, with a drop from 88% of younger women to 34% of those in the older age group. Amongst older women, Gujerati and Punjabi (G) are also mentioned by sizeable minorities. However, in this group, 25% are unable to read any of the languages covered in the survey.

Amongst Pakistanis English is the most frequently mentioned language of literacy (63%) followed closely by Urdu (56%). A further 12% mentioned Punjabi in the Urdu script. A total of 17% report not to be able to read any of their languages covered. Amongst women, the level of illiteracy rises dramatically from 11% of younger women to 68% of those aged 50 to 74.

Of the three South Asian communities, Bangladeshis report the lowest rates of literacy in English (52%). However, almost four in five (79%) report to be literate in Bengali. Subsequently, illiteracy for the community as a whole is 11%. Again, it is older women where lack of literacy is more pronounced (52%). With the exception of this group, literacy in Bengali is high across all the age and gender sub-groups. By contrast, literacy in English declines significantly across age groups; for women from 64% of younger women to 4% of those in the older group, and for men from 90% of the younger age group to 38% of the older one.

Table 7: Languages read (Source: AS Q20)

Ethnic group	Language	All %	Women 16–29 %	Women 30–49 %	Women 50–74 %	Men 16–29 %	Men 30-49 %	Men 50–74 %
Indian	English	76	88	67	34	96	83	71
	Gujerati	34	27	42	31	14	43	47
	Punjabi (G)	21	22	21	24	12	28	21
	Hindi	18	14	17	20	7	28	21
	Urdu	8	8	6	5	3	10	17
	Punjabi (U)	5	5	5	4	3	4	10
	None	5	0	4	25	0	2	6
Pakistani	English	63	77	31	7	91	77	54
	Urdu	56	55	50	17	53	70	69
	Punjabi (U)	12	4	15	3	15	13	17
	None	17	11	31	68	1	7	16
Bangladeshi	Bengali	79	87	74	43	81	88	78
	English	52	64	15	4	90	60	38
	None	11	0	24	52	0	3	19

Base: All adults

Table 8 shows which language is the preferred reading language for each of the three South Asian communities. Amongst Indians, English is mentioned by just over half (52%). Not surprisingly, it is young women (75%) and men (87%) who are particularly likely to mention English. Gujerati is mentioned by a further 24%, and Punjabi (G) by 12%. Both of these languages gain in importance amongst those aged 30 or over. Only 2% mention Hindi as their preferred language of literacy. This raises questions about the benefits of providing translations in Hindi, which is very frequently included in the production of written materials aimed at South Asian communities.

Amongst Pakistanis, the youngest age band identifies English as their preferred language of literacy. After age 30 however, Urdu is the preferred medium for written communications. Although there is a written version of Punjabi (U) only 5% report this to be a preferred written medium.

Written Bengali is a stated preference of 60% of Bangladeshis. Just over a quarter (27%) identify English as their preferred reading language. For both older Bangladeshi and Pakistani women, the high illiteracy rates limit the possibilities for written communications.

Table 8: Preferred reading language (Source: AS Q21)

Ethnic group	Language	All %	Women 16–29 %	Women 30–49 %	Women 50–74 %	Men 16–29 %	Men 30–49 %	Men 50–74 %
Indian	English	52	75	36	16	87	53	29
	Gujerati	24	18	35	29	8	26	31
	Punjabi (G)	12	6	16	16	2	14	18
	Hindi	2	0	2	9	0	1	3
	Illiterate	5	0	4	25	0	2	6
Pakistani	English	40	63	7	0	76	37	12
	Urdu	33	21	46	17	16	47	58
	Punjabi (U)	5	2	10	2	4	4	7
	Illiterate	17	11	31	68	1	7	18
Bangladeshi	Bengali	60	57	73	43	38	77	74
	English	27	42	1	0	62	19	4
	Illiterate	11	0	24	52	0	3	19

Base: All adults

As we have pointed out above, answers to the questions about spoken and written language in this survey are all based on respondents' own assessment. The survey did include a question asking respondents to scale their level of literacy in English (see Table 9). This table shows a considerable gradient in the perceived ability to read English amongst those who previously reported that they can read English (see Table 7).

For Indians, high proportions report that they can read English very well (47%). A further 20% report that they can read English fairly well or a little. The ratio between those who report they can read very well and only fairly well/a little is much closer for Pakistanis and Bangladeshis. For the first group, 31% report that they can read English very well, compared to 26% who can read fairly well/a little; for Bangladeshis the ratio is 1 with 24% falling into either category. In other words, competence (based on self-assessment) is higher amongst Indians and lower amongst Bangladeshis.

Table 9: Self-rated level of literacy in English (Source: AS Q23)

			Read English			
		Very well	Fairly well	A little	Do not read (Q20)	Don't know No answer
Ethnic group	Sub-group	%	%	%	%	%
Indian	All	47	14	6	24	9
	Women: 16–29	64	12	3	12	9
	30–49	35	17	7	33	8
	50–74	19	4	10	66	1
	Men: 16–29	68	10	1	4	17
	30–49	49	19	6	17	9
	50–74	31	16	14	29	10
Pakistani	All	31	21	5	37	6
	Women: 16–29	44	21	4	23	8
	30–49	11	13	5	69	3
	50–74	0	2	2	93	0
	Men: 16–29	51	24	3	9	13
	30–49	31	35	9	23	2
	50–74	24	21	7	46	2
Bangladeshi	All	24	15	9	48	4
	Women: 16–29	39	13	7	36	5
	30–49	2	2	8	85	3
	50–74	0	2	2	96	0
	Men: 16–29	53	24	6	10	7
	30–49	14	26	15	40	5
	50–74	6	14	18	62	0

Base: All adults

Work status

Table 10 shows the work status of the populations sampled in this survey. Comparisons are made with the UK-wide 1992 Health and Lifestyles Survey, with the target audience aged 16 to 74, and also with the Census data for 16 to 65 year olds, shown in Table 11.

Firstly, comparing the UK average in Table 10, with the Census average in Table 11, it can be seen that there is a very close correspondence between the survey figures and the Census figures, with two exceptions: firstly, full-time employment rates are 7% higher in the Census, and secondly, the proportion of retired people is 9% lower in the Census. Bearing in mind that the survey population included 66 to 74 year olds (who are not included in the Census statistic), the work status statistics show a very close match between the survey population and the Census population for the national Health and Lifestyles Survey.

There is however greater variation when comparing the work status figures for the current survey respondents, and the Census (this may partially be attributable to the longer time gap between the survey and the Census). Again, the proportions registered as being in full-time work in the Census are significantly higher than was found in the survey. This survey also shows significantly higher rates of unemployment, especially amongst African-Caribbeans and Bangladeshis, than the Census. For example, the Census reports a 15% unemployment rate for 16 to 65 year old African-Caribbeans; the figure found in the survey was 23%. For Bangladeshis, the Census unemployment rate was 16%, compared to 22% in the survey. Since the survey focused on ethnic minorities living in urban areas, it is likely that the communities covered in the survey sampling strategy are marginally more deprived than the total ethnic minority population. However, other comparisons such as those for household tenure (Tables 14 and 15) show that tenure profiles are very similar between both sources. The exception is the Bangladeshi community, which in the survey has a higher incidence of local authority housing and of housing association rented accommodation.

Table 10: Respondents' work status (Source: AS Q28; AC Q33)

	All adults				UK population %
	African-Caribbean %	Indian %	Pakistani %	Bangladeshi %	
Employee, full-time	33	35	20	16	40
Employee, part-time	6	6	3	2	12
Self-employed	3	6	4	2	6
Unemployed (less than 6 months)	6	2	4	4	2
Unemployed (more than 6 months)	17	11	13	18	5
Sick, disabled (less than 6 months)	0	1	<0.05	1	<0.05
Sick, disabled (more than 6 months)	5	4	6	4	3
Full-time education	9	10	12	14	12
Retired	9	5	5	3	6
Looking after home/family	10	19	31	34	13

Base: All adults

Table 11: Census analysis of work status (Source: OPCS)

	All adults				UK population %
	African-Caribbean %	Indian %	Pakistani %	Bangladeshi %	
Full-time work	50	42	24	23	47
Part-time work	8	6	3	3	12
Self-employed	4	12	9	6	8
Unemployed	15	9	15	16	7
Permanently sick	5	10	12	12	5
Retired	5	4	6	6	4
Full-time education	3	2	1	1	4
Other	10	15	30	33	13

Base: All adults

Table 12a shows the employment status for women from the four different ethnic minority communities, and for the women represented in the UK-wide Health and Lifestyles Survey. Full-time employment rates for African-Caribbean women are higher, and for Indian women the same, as the UK average. There is, however, very little full-time work amongst Pakistani or Bangladeshi women.

Whilst one in five women throughout the UK work part-time, the proportion amongst African-Caribbeans and Indians is half that size; there are negligible rates of part-time working amongst Pakistani and Bangladeshi women.

Unemployment rates are significantly higher amongst African-Caribbean women and are also marginally higher amongst Indian and Pakistani women.

The most pronounced differences amongst the four community groups can be found in the category of 'looking after home/family'. The figures for the UK average, and for African-Caribbean women are very similar (23% and 19% respectively). Amongst Indian women, the proportion who look after the home/family rises to 38%. By contrast, the vast majority of Pakistani women (64%) and Bangladeshi women (70%) classify themselves as looking after the home/family full-time.

One other noticeable difference is that the rate of women in full-time education is roughly twice as high for each of the ethnic minority groups as for the UK as a whole.

Table 12a: Women's work status (Source: AS Q28; AC Q33)

	All women				UK population
	African-Caribbean %	Indian %	Pakistani %	Bangladeshi %	%
Employee, full-time	34	26	6	5	26
Employee, part-time	10	9	3	2	21
Self-employed	1	3	<0.5	0	5
Unemployed (less than 6 months)	3	1	1	1	1
Unemployed (more than 6 months)	12	6	5	4	3
Sick, disabled (less than 6 months)	0	1	0	0	<0.5
Sick, disabled (more than 6 months)	4	3	5	<0.5	2
Looking after home/family	19	38	64	70	23
Full-time education	10	9	11	12	5
Retired	6	4	3	1	13

Base: All women

Table 12b shows the matching employment data for men. Employment rates amongst all of the ethnic groups covered in the survey are signicantly lower than those for the comparable UK sample. In the UK sample, a total of 10% of men classified themselves as unemployed. By contrast, amongst Indian men the figure is 21%, amongst Pakistani men 27%, amongst African-Caribbean men 32%, and amongst Bangladeshi men 37%.

Again, a higher proportion of men from all four communities describe themselves as being in full-time education.

South Asian men, particularly Bangladeshis, show above average rates of sickness or disability.

Table 12b: Men's work status (Source: AS Q28; AC Q33)

	All men				UK population %
	African-Caribbean %	Indian %	Pakistani %	Bangladeshi %	
Employee, full-time	33	44	33	25	54
Employee, part-time	1	4	3	2	2
Self-employed	4	9	8	3	9
Unemployed (less than 6 months)	9	4	6	7	3
Unemployed (more than 6 months)	23	17	21	30	7
Sick, disabled (less than 6 months)	0	<0.5	<0.5	2	<0.5
Sick, disabled (more than 6 months)	6	5	7	8	3
Looking after home/family	1	1	1	2	1
Full-time education	9	10	13	17	6
Retired	12	6	6	3	14

Base: All men

It must be borne in mind, however, that the Labour Force Survey surveys a slightly younger population, and that in addition, no mother-tongue interviewing was provided. It therefore seems likely that the difference in reported educational attainment between the current survey and the PSI analysis of the Labour Force Survey (Jones, 1993) is most likely to be the result of these sampling and methodological differences.

Table 13a: Educational status of respondent (Source: AS Q31a,b; AC Q39)

UK qualifications	Women				Men				UK population	
	African-Caribbean %	Indian %	Pakis-tani %	Bangla-deshi %	African-Caribbean %	Indian %	Pakis-tani %	Bangla-deshi %	Women %	Men %
Degree or higher	2	2	2	1	2	5	4	3	5	6
Professional qualification	1	1	1	<0.5	1	1	1	1	2	5
Higher education/ below degree level	11	4	3	2	3	5	5	2	8	7
GCE A level or equivalent	14	11	6	5	21	13	9	7	18	28
GCE O level or equivalent	28	19	17	14	25	15	14	16	23	18
Any UK qualification	62	41	32	23	60	45	39	32	63	71
No UK qualification	38	59	68	77	40	55	61	68	37	29
Any foreign qualifications	NA	24	20	22	NA	28	32	25	–	–
– degree/ professional qualification	–	5	2	1	–	5	7	3	–	–

Education

Table 13a shows the highest educational qualifications obtained by respondents. The table shows UK qualifications; in addition for South Asians it shows the proportions who obtained qualifications in other countries.

When comparing women first, it can be seen that the professional and educational qualifications of African-Caribbean women and the UK average are broadly similar. Although only 3% of African-Caribbean women have degrees or professional qualifications (compared with 7% of the UK average obtained from the UK-wide Health and Lifestyles Survey), 11% hold higher educational qualifications below degree level (compared to 8% for the UK average).

For Indian women the proportion who hold degrees, professional qualifications or other higher educational qualifications obtained in the UK declines to 7% (compared to 15% for the UK average). However, a further 5% hold degrees or professional qualifications obtained abroad. GCE A level or O level equivalents also are mentioned less frequently and, not surprisingly, significantly higher proportions hold no UK qualifications at all (59% versus 37%).

Among Pakistani and Bangladeshi women, lower proportions hold degree or professional qualifications (8% and 4% respectively). The proportion who hold no UK qualifications rises to 68% and 77% respectively.

Amongst men from black and minority ethnic communities, those classified as Indian and Pakistani have the highest rates of degree, professional, or higher educational qualifications (11% and 10% respectively, compared to a UK average of 18%). A further 5% of Indian men and 7% of Pakistani men have similar qualifications obtained abroad.

Higher-level qualifications are mentioned less frequently by Bangladeshi men and by African-Caribbean men.

Overall, 29% of men in the UK-wide Health and Lifestyles Survey had no UK educational qualifications; amongst African-Caribbean men this rises to 40%, and amongst Indian men to 55%. The highest rates are found for Pakistani (61%), and Bangladeshi men (68%).

The comparison with the Labour Force Survey shows a number of variations. For example, significantly higher levels of degree or higher qualifications are reported in the Labour Force Survey (Table 13b). There are also differences in the educational qualifications reported in the other attainment bands. It must be remembered that the Labour Force Survey did not offer any mother-tongue interviewing.

Table 13b: Labour Force Survey: highest educational qualification (Source: PSI)

UK qualifications	Women				Men				UK population	
	African-Caribbean %	Indian %	Pakis-tani %	Bangla-deshi %	African-Caribbean %	Indian %	Pakis-tani %	Bangla-deshi %	Women %	Men %
Degree or higher	3	9	3	4	4	15	5	7	6	10
Higher education/ below degree level	13	5	1	1	2	4	2	0	7	5
GCE A level or equivalent	16	9	4	2	31	19	13	5	14	33
GCE O level or equivalent	19	14	8	8	12	9	8	8	22	12
Any UK qualification	69	55	31	24	65	66	48	39	64	72
No UK qualification	31	45	69	76	35	34	52	61	36	28

Housing

Table 14 shows the household tenure data for the four target audiences, and the UK comparison. Amongst the UK-wide Health and Lifestyles Survey, 74% are owner-occupiers. Slightly higher rates are found for Indians (85%) and Pakistanis (81%). Owner-occupancy is lowest amongst African-Caribbeans (51%) and Bangladeshis (33%). Amongst these two groups, much higher proportions live in local authority housing (34% of African-Caribbeans, and 49% of Bangladeshis). It is also noticeable that very low proportions of Indians and Pakistanis live in local authority housing (6% and 5% respectively, compared to 17% for the UK population).

Table 15 shows the same figures derived from the 1991 Census. It must be remembered that the Census figures cover an older population (the age cut-off for survey participation was 74 years). For the UK averages, the two data sources show a remarkably close correspondence. There is however more diversion for the different ethnic minority communities. In the main this centres around the higher proportions reporting to own their households outright in the survey, than in the Census. By contrast, fewer report to be buying on a mortgage in the survey than in the Census. However, when aggregating the two owner-occupier figures, the overall classification of owner-occupier is identical across the two data sources for African-Caribbeans, Indians, and Pakistanis. As mentioned earlier, the remaining significant difference is for Bangladeshis, where this survey records a higher proportion living in local authority or housing association accommodation, and a lower proportion of owner-occupiers. Overall, we would conclude that the match between the survey and the Census (as far as household tenure is concern) is very good. The exception is the sample of Bangladeshis, which is skewed towards the local authority housing sector.

Table 14: Household tenure (Source: AS Q4; AC Q4)

	All adults				UK population %
	African-Caribbean %	Indian %	Pakistani %	Bangladeshi %	
Own outright	21	38	37	11	24
Buying on mortgage	30	47	44	22	50
Rent from council	34	6	5	49	17
Rent from housing association	9	3	3	12	2
Rent from private landlord	6	6	10	7	5

Base: All adults

Table 15: Census analysis of household tenure (Source: OPCS)

	All adults				UK population %
	African-Caribbean %	Indian %	Pakistani %	Bangladeshi %	
Own outright	8	18	21	5	20
Buying on mortgage	44	68	60	39	51
Rent from council	34	6	9	40	18
Rent from housing association	8	2	2	6	2
Rent from private landlord	4	5	7	8	6

Base: All adults

Further information about the type of housing different communities live in is shown in Table 16. The housing environment differs significantly from the UK average. Amongst Bangladeshis almost half live in flats (46%), compared to a UK average of 8%. The predominant housing environment for Indians and Pakistanis are mid-terraces (62% and 67% respectively, compared to a UK average of 20%).

Table 16: Type of housing (Source: AS Q8/9; AC Q13/14)

	All adults				UK population %
	African-Caribbean %	Indian %	Pakistani %	Bangladeshi %	
House/bungalow					
– detached	2	4	2	1	25
– semi-detached/ end terrace	19	25	21	9	45
– mid terrace	41	62	67	35	20
Maisonette	7	1	1	5	1
Flat	28	6	4	46	8
Room/bedsitter	1	<0.5	1	1	<0.5

Base: All adults

Table 17 shows that identical or even higher proportions of African-Caribbeans, Bangladeshis, and Indians have use of mains gas central heating than the UK average. Only Pakistanis report a lower rate of centrally heated housing; for this group, gas fires are the predominant form of heating (63%).

Table 17: Form of heating used (Source: AS Q7; AC Q12)

	All adults				UK population %
	African-Caribbean %	Indian %	Pakistani %	Bangladeshi %	
Central heating					
– mains gas	71	81	50	72	67
– electric/normal tariff	5	3	3	3	2
– electric/off-peak	3	1	<0.5	1	4
Non-central heating					
– mains gas	25	37	61	38	27
– electric bar fire	5	4	8	6	8
– fan heater	3	4	5	4	3
– calor/butane gas	3	1	2	<0.5	3

Base: All adults

Table 18 compares access to cars amongst the different black and minority ethnic communities. In the UK-wide Health and Lifestyles Survey, 59% of respondents hold a driving licence and also own a car. A further 4% hold a licence and have access to a car. The remainder either do not have a driving licence or access to a car.

The comparison with the black and minority ethnic communities reveals striking differences. The highest rate of access to a car is found amongst Indians, where 41% have both a driver's licence and car and a further 3% have access to a car. Amongst Pakistanis, the respective figures are 29% and 2% and amongst African-Caribbeans 26% and 3%. The Bangladeshi community shows the lowest rate of car ownership and access to a car. Here, only 16% have both a car and a driver's licence, and only a further 2% who hold a licence have access to a car.

Table 18: Access to car (Source: AS Q10/11; AC Q15/16)

	All adults				UK population %
	African-Caribbean %	Indian %	Pakistani %	Bangladeshi %	
Own car/have driver's licence	26	41	29	16	60
Access to car/have driver's licence	3	3	2	2	4
No car/have driver's licence	11	8	8	9	5
No licence	60	48	61	73	30

Base: All adults

3. Perceptions of health

Health status

This survey included a number of questions inviting participants to describe their health status. It must be recognised that these are subjective responses, but at the same time that they also provide some broad indicators of the prevalence of poorer health status, as well as some predictors of likely uptake of health services (Blaxter, 1985; 1990). The question formats used have been well established in successive General Household Surveys. The format used for the UK-wide Health and Lifestyles Survey was identical to that used in the General Household Survey. The surveys of black and minority ethnic communities, which followed later, used an amended question wording. The piloting work for the black and minority ethnic groups survey showed that the concept of 'longstanding' illness, and the phrase ' limit your activities in any way' were difficult to comprehend both in the English and mother-tongue versions. It was therefore necessary to simplify the question wording for the current survey. We will return to the possible implications of this deviation later.

A possibly useful source for national comparisons would have been the 1991 Census. This included a question on health status, but the question wording again was signifi-cantly different from that used in the General Household Survey. As a result, the reported prevalence of limiting long-term illness in the Census is 11.5% (for 16–74 year olds), compared to the figure for limiting longstanding illness, obtained in the General Household Survey of 1989, of 18.5% for the same age band.

It is therefore not possible to draw meaningful comparisons between the results obtained for the ethnic minority groups covered in the Census, and those obtained in the current survey, because of these differences in question wording.

Table 19 shows the first of the health status assessments used in the survey. Results are presented in two forms: firstly, the results for each ethnic group, weighted to the Census characteristics of that particular population group. Throughout the remainder of the report these findings are shown under the overall headings of 'All adults'.

Secondly, the findings have been weighted to the age and sex profile of the UK population. This age/sex standardisation removes the effects of any age or gender imbalances between a particular ethnic minority population and the UK population at large. It should be noted at this point that the standardisation only had a minor impact on the overall findings. Whilst the age profiles of the different minority ethnic groups are significantly different from that of the white population, most of these differences occur around the extremes of the age dimensions. For example, around 40% of the South Asian population is aged under 16, compared to around 20% of the white population. Similarly, one in five of the white population are of retirement age, compared to around one in twenty of the Asian population. But within the age bands covered in this survey (16–74 year olds) the discrepancies between the different populations are less marked. For this reason, the age/sex standardisations did not have a dramatic impact. Unless stated otherwise, we therefore comment on the findings obtained for each ethnic group, rather than the standardised figures.

The UK-wide Health and Lifestyles Survey showed that 47% of the adult population (16–74 year olds) define their health status as very good, and a further 45% describe it as fairly good. Six per cent describe their health status as fairly poor, and 2% as very poor. There are some significant differences in the proportions of members of the different minority ethnic communities who describe their health status as very or fairly poor. Amongst African-Caribbeans, a total of 14% describe their health status as poor; amongst Indians, this figure rises to 17%, and amongst Pakistanis to 20%. The proportion who describe their health status as poor is particularly high amongst Bangladeshis, with 27% describing their health status as very or fairly poor.

Table 19: Perceived health status (Source: AS Q32; AC Q40)

Health status	All adults				Standardised				UK population
	African-Caribbean	Indian	Pakis-tani	Bangla-deshi	African-Caribbean	Indian	Pakis-tani	Bangla-deshi	
	%	%	%	%	%	%	%	%	%
Very good	43	45	37	35	39	45	38	34	47
Fairly good	43	39	43	38	44	39	43	36	45
Fairly poor	8	11	14	18	9	11	14	20	6
Very poor	6	6	6	9	8	5	6	10	2

Base: All adults

Table 20 shows in greater detail the proportions of the various population sub-groups who describe their health status as very or fairly poor. As one would expect, for all ethnic groups there is an increase in this figure with increasing age. It is noticeable, however that the rate of this increase is much more pronounced amongst South Asians.

Table 20: Proportion who describe health status as poor (Source: AS Q32; AC Q40)

Demographic group	All adults				Standardised				UK population %
	African-Caribbean %	Indian %	Pakis-tani %	Bangla-deshi %	African-Caribbean %	Indian %	Pakis-tani %	Bangla-deshi %	
All	14	17	20	28	17	16	20	29	8
Women	13	17	24	27	16	17	21	30	8
16–29	7	5	13	6	8	7	11	6	4
30–49	10	11	28	45	10	11	25	48	6
50–74	30	52	52	55	29	48	53	55	12
Men	14	16	16	28	19	16	18	29	7
16–29	4	6	9	6	4	5	10	7	3
30–49	4	16	13	21	4	15	15	21	4
50–74	37	33	34	64	38	34	35	65	15

Base: All adults

Table 21 shows the answers to the first of a set of questions used in the General Household Survey to measure the prevalence of limiting longstanding illness and disability. As mentioned above, the question wording for the South Asian questionnaires differed from that used for the UK-wide survey and for the survey of African-Caribbeans. But as the follow-on question itemising the specific illnesses and diseases (e.g. hypertension, diabetes, asthma, etc.) referred to shows (see Table 22), there appears to be consistent evidence suggesting that the higher subjective expression of poor health amongst South Asians has an underlying epidemiology.

Overall, there is no difference in current self-reported illness or disability between the UK population and the African-Caribbean and Indian population. Reported rates are higher amongst Pakistanis and peak amongst Bangladeshis. Even when allowing for the relatively small cell sizes for some of the demographic sub-groups, the higher rates of reported problems amongst older South Asian women are significant. Amongst Bangladeshis, there also appears to be a high rate of reported illness amongst women aged 30 to 49, whilst the highest rate is recorded for older Bangladeshi men.

Table 21: Prevalence of illness or disability (Source: AS Q33/34a; AC Q41/42a)

Demographic group	All adults				Standardised				
	African-Caribbean %	Indian %	Pakis-tani %	Bangla-deshi %	African-Caribbean %	Indian %	Pakis-tani %	Bangla-deshi %	UK population %
All	26	27	31	35	29	26	30	36	27
Women	26	29	32	32	28	27	30	35	28
16–29	22	13	20	10	22	12	18	10	17
30–49	18	25	37	50	17	24	34	52	24
50–74	47	70	61	60	46	67	61	60	42
Men	26	25	30	38	31	25	31	38	27
16–29	8	8	20	11	8	9	19	12	15
30–49	29	24	26	34	28	23	28	34	21
50–74	47	51	56	78	48	52	55	77	38

Base: All adults

The survey included an open-ended question aimed at assessing the illness or problem referred to by respondents. The coding of answers to this question followed the format established for the General Household Survey. Table 22 shows the difference in current reported illnesses or problems between the UK population and each of the black and minority ethnic communities. Key differences can be found in the reported prevalence of hypertension, diabetes, and for Bangladeshis, in digestive problems, including stomach ulcers. Evidence for ethnic variations in mortality risk from hypertensive diseases is well established (e.g. Cruickshank, 1993; OPCS, 1990). Similarly, the work by McKeigue and Marmot (1991) and Cruickshank et al. (1991) demonstrates significantly higher rates of non-insulin dependent diabetes amongst South Asians than amongst Europeans.

Table 22: Illness/diseases mentioned frequently (Source: AS Q34a; AC Q42a)

	All adults				UK population %
	African-Caribbean %	Indian %	Pakistani %	Bangladeshi %	
Any	26	27	31	35	28
Hypertension/high blood pressure	4	5	2	5	2
Asthma	2	4	5	4	3
Arthritis/rheumatism /fibrositis	3	4	4	2	5
Diabetes	2	4	4	7	1
Back problems/slipped disc	3	3	5	2	3
Other back problems	1	2	3	6	1
Other problems of the bones/joints	1	2	2	4	3
Other digestive problems	1	1	2	5	1
Other respiratory problems	1	2	2	2	1
Migraine/headaches	1	1	2	3	1
Mental illness/anxiety	1	1	2	1	1
Stomach ulcers/abdominal hernia	1	<0.5	1	3	1

Base: All adults

Apart from the open-ended questions about current illnesses or health problems reported on above, respondents were also shown a list of problems or diseases (those who could not read were read the list) and were asked if they had ever experienced any of them. Table 23 shows the reported experiences of the various illnesses or symptoms for each of the ethnic groups, compared with the national average obtained from the UK-wide Health and Lifestyles Survey.

The differences between the black and minority ethnic communities and the white population are less pronounced in this table. For example, very similar proportions report respiratory problems, or refer to heart disease. There is less reference to depression or other mental health problems amongst all of the minority ethnic communities. High blood pressure is mentioned most frequently by African-Caribbeans, but is reported less frequently by South Asians, when compared to the UK average. Bangladeshis again report a much higher occurrence of stomach problems. Across all the minority ethnic communities, diabetes is reported more frequently than by the UK population.

Table 23: Experience of specific health problems (Source: AS Q36; AC Q50)

	All adults				Standardised				
	African-Caribbean %	Indian %	Pakis-tani %	Bangla-deshi %	African-Caribbean %	Indian %	Pakis-tani %	Bangla-deshi %	UK population %
Back pain	25	20	24	20	26	21	23	20	29
Breathing difficulties (e.g. bronchitis)	11	9	12	11	11	9	11	11	11
Severe arthritis/ rheumatism	8	8	9	13	10	8	7	13	10
Depression/anxiety nerves	7	8	9	5	7	7	8	6	14
High blood pressure	12	8	8	9	16	8	8	10	14
Stomach problems (e.g. ulcers)	5	6	9	14	6	6	8	14	NA
Diabetes	5	6	5	8	5	5	6	8	2
Heart disease	2	3	4	6	2	2	3	5	3
Thalassaemia	<0.5	1	1	<0.5	<0.5	1	1	<0.5	NA
Stroke	2	1	<0.5	1	2	1	1	<0.5	1
Sexually transmitted diseases	1	1	0	0	1	<0.5	0	0	<0.5
Anorexia nervosa	0	1	<0.5	<0.5	0	<0.5	<0.5	<0.5	1
Alcoholism	0	<0.5	1	<0.5	0	<0.5	<0.5	<0.5	<0.5
Sickle cell	2	<0.5	<0.5	<0.5	2	1	0	<0.5	NA
Any of listed problems	56	44	49	47	59	45	47	48	56

Base: All adults

Table 24, the final table in this set of findings, shows the reported prevalence of limiting illnesses or disabilities. Again, it must be emphasised that the question wording used for the South Asian questionnaires differed from that used for the UK survey and for African-Caribbeans. However, the same overall pattern of the more widespread reporting of illness or health problems amongst Bangladeshis, and amongst older South Asian women can be found.

Table 24: Prevalence of limiting illness or disability (Source: AS Q33/34b; AC Q41/42b)

Demographic group	All adults				Standardised				UK population
	African-Caribbean %	Indian %	Pakis-tani %	Bangla-deshi %	African-Caribbean %	Indian %	Pakis-tani %	Bangla-deshi %	%
All	17	17	21	25	20	16	20	26	15
Women	16	18	19	24	18	16	20	26	16
16–29	11	5	12	6	12	6	10	6	9
30–49	11	15	25	40	11	15	25	41	13
50–74	32	50	45	43	31	40	43	41	26
Men	17	16	22	26	21	16	20	26	14
16–29	6	4	12	5	6	4	12	6	6
30–49	13	14	17	23	13	12	18	23	10
50–74	37	38	43	57	37	38	38	55	27

Base: All adults

Risk factors

The questionnaire included a detailed question about which risk factors people felt had a negative effect on their health at the moment. For those who could read, these risk factors were shown on a showcard, whilst those who were unable to read had the factors read out to them by the interviewer. Again, Table 25 shows comparisons between the UK-wide Health and Lifestyles Survey, and the surveys of the different black and minority ethnic communities.

The table groups factors under three broad headings: firstly, lifestyle factors, secondly psycho-social factors, and thirdly a broad category of other factors, mainly consisting of environmental factors. For the UK population, lifestyle factors are seen as the major health risks. For example, 24% mentioned their weight as having a bad effect on their health at the moment, 18% mentioned the amount they smoke, and 15% the kind of food they eat. Concern about weight is of less importance to most of the black and minority ethnic communities. Similarly, lower proportions mention the amount they smoke. As Chapter 5 shows, smoking rates amongst the different black and minority ethnic communities are lower than amongst the white population. However, even amongst those who do smoke, smoking is less likely to be identified as a health risk.

For the set of categories on psycho-social health, a slightly different question wording had to be adopted for the South Asian questionnaires. Here, the concept of 'stress' could not be transferred easily into the South Asian cultures, and a more acceptable phrase of 'worries' had to be used. The figures shown in Table 25 would suggest that stress or worries at home are a significant concern especially to Pakistanis and Bangladeshis.

Table 25 also shows that significant proportions of members of the different communities feel that their health is negatively affected by social and environmental factors. As Chapter 2 shows, unemployment rates are significantly higher and it is therefore not surprising that larger proportions consider unemployment has a poor effect on their health. High proportions also are concerned about the amount of violent crime in the area in which they live. When comparing these figures with the UK figures it must be borne in mind that the black and minority ethnic community data refer to urban neighbourhoods.

The perceived impact of racism is also worthy of comment. The proportions who feel it has a poor effect on their health are similar to those who refer to smoking or exercise.

The single most frequently mentioned health risk by any of the different target groups is the effect of poor housing identified by the Bangladeshi community. Table 26 provides more detailed information about this phenomenon.

Table 25: Factors perceived to have a bad effect on health at the moment (Source: AS Q35; AC Q47)

	All adults				Standardised				
	African-Caribbean %	Indian %	Pakis-tani %	Bangla-deshi %	African-Caribbean %	Indian %	Pakis-tani %	Bangla-deshi %	UK population %
Lifestyle factors									
My weight	18	15	15	7	18	16	13	7	24
The amount I smoke	13	3	6	7	12	3	6	6	18
The kind of food I eat	11	12	13	11	10	11	12	11	15
The amount of exercise I do	10	5	6	2	9	5	5	2	NA
The amount of alcohol I drink	3	2	1	<0.5	3	2	1	<0.5	5
My sexual behaviour	1	<0.5	1	1	1	<0.5	1	1	1
Psycho-social factors									
Stress/worries at work	13	5	3	1	12	5	3	1	17
Stress/worries at at home	12	11	16	17	14	12	16	17	9
Living on my own	5	2	2	1	6	2	2	1	3
Social/environmental									
Environmental pollution in general	21	12	6	7	19	9	5	6	15
Being unemployed	17	10	11	14	15	9	11	13	6
The amount of violent crime in this area	15	15	14	18	15	14	13	17	6
Environmental pollution where I live	12	8	6	7	11	7	6	6	6
Road traffic in this area	9	10	9	4	10	10	8	4	8
Quality of my housing	8	5	11	27	8	5	11	26	2
The amount of racism in this area	6	6	8	8	5	6	7	7	1
Environmental pollution where I live	5	5	2	1	4	4	2	1	5
Any risk factor	78	59	61	68	77	57	58	67	73

Base: All adults

As mentioned above, concerns about the quality of housing are top of the Bangladeshi community's concerns about potential health risk. The questionnaire explored in more detail which aspects of the housing environment are perceived to be a potential health risk. As the last row in Table 26 shows, almost half of the UK population identifies housing-related variables as having a potential risk on their health. Amongst African-Caribbeans, this figures rises to 68%, and amongst Bangladeshis to 84%.

Amongst the UK population at large, concerns about the quality of drinking water are the most frequently mentioned item. Whilst this is also a concern to African-Caribbeans, amongst this group other housing-related concerns feature. For example, almost one in five identify dampness, noise levels, lack of heating, or lack of space as problematic. Pakistanis also identify dampness and lack of heating as a potential health risk; it should be remembered that this group had the lowest central heating installation rates.

The group for whom housing variables are of greatest concern are Bangladeshis. Over four in five expressed a concern about housing variables. Specific concerns include 40% who feel their health is at risk from dampness, 35% who mention lack of space, and 26% who mention lack of heating or general maintenance of their home. A further 25% are concerned about condensation, and 18% about mould. It must be remembered that large proportions of this population group live in flats provided by local authorities. The work on housing-related health problems amongst Bangladeshis in the East End of London provides some illustration of the specific problems faced by this community (Hyndman, 1990).

Table 26: Perceived risk to health in home (Source: AS Q37c; AC Q53)

	All adults				Standardised				
	African-Caribbean %	Indian %	Pakistani %	Bangladeshi %	African-Caribbean %	Indian %	Pakistani %	Bangladeshi %	UK population %
Quality of drinking water	23	11	7	3	21	9	5	3	22
Dampness	19	15	24	40	18	17	26	40	7
Lack of sound proofing/level of noise	19	9	10	15	16	8	10	15	9
Lack of heating	18	8	15	26	18	10	16	26	6
Lack of personal space/not enough space	17	9	15	35	15	10	14	33	7
General maintenance of home	16	8	11	26	15	8	12	25	7
Condensation	13	11	11	25	14	12	12	25	6
Mould	5	4	4	18	6	4	5	17	3
Any risk factor	68	47	54	84	66	45	52	73	45

Base: All adults

Involvement in health-enhancing activities

The survey tried to assess to what extent people feel they are engaged in activities which either maintain or improve their health. The question was followed up with an open-ended question to assess what kind of activities people actually consider to be health-maintaining or health-enhancing. Answers include a very large number of individual sports, general physical activities, such as gardening, attending health clinics, changes in dietary behaviour, the use of dietary supplements, the taking of medication, etc.

In total, 62% of the UK population feel they are involved in some kind of health-maintaining or health-enhancing activity (see Table 27). Figures for all the minority ethnic communities show much lower rates of participation. Amongst African-Caribbeans, 55% report to be involved in such activities, amongst Indians 46%, amongst Bangladeshis 37%, and amongst Pakistanis 41%. Whilst amongst the national population there is no difference between men and women, women from the minority ethnic communities are much less likely to report any involvement in health-enhancing activities.

Table 27: Involvement in health-enhancing activities (Source: AS Q34c; AC Q43)

| Demographic group | All adults | | | | Standardised | | | | |
	African-Caribbean %	Indian %	Pakis-tani %	Bangla-deshi %	African-Caribbean %	Indian %	Pakis-tani %	Bangla-deshi %	UK population %
All	55	46	41	37	53	43	38	37	62
Women	52	38	33	29	51	35	30	31	61
16–29	48	37	31	27	48	36	29	28	62
30–49	59	33	30	29	57	31	28	32	58
50+	45	50	43	38	46	42	42	38	64
Men	60	54	49	45	56	52	46	43	63
16–29	65	61	62	59	61	61	59	58	67
30–49	63	50	39	33	63	48	38	33	61
50+	48	53	44	36	48	46	35	34	61

Base: All adults

Table 28 shows the proportion of each population group engaged in health-enhancing activities. In the table the activities are grouped into broad categories. Firstly, there are figures for the involvement in any specific activity. The second band of results shows involvement in sports-based activities. The third band of findings, entitled 'General physical activity', covers non-sports-based activities such as walking, do-it-yourself, gardening, etc. The fourth band entitled 'Diet' includes any reference to dietary changes or improvements.

We also found significant proportions mentioning medication, and these references are grouped together under the fifth heading of 'Medical treatment'. Finally, the sixth heading covers any other lifestyle modifications such as reduction in alcohol intake or smoking reduction or cessation.

In the UK-wide Health and Lifestyles Survey, 39% of the population mention sports-based activities. The proportion mentioning such activities amongst the different black and minority ethnic communities is significantly lower. Amongst African-Caribbeans and Indians, 30% and 29% respectively mention such activities. Amongst Pakistanis the figure falls to 24%, and amongst Bangladeshis it falls even further to 20%.

Sports-based activity is mentioned slightly more frequently by men than women in the UK-wide survey, and mentions decrease with age. The gender difference for the black and minority ethnic communities is much more pronounced. For example, just over a quarter of African-Caribbean and Indian women aged 16 to 29 mention sports-based activities; amongst young Pakistani and Bangladeshi women this falls to 17%, compared to a UK average figure of 50% for the matching age and gender band.

Other forms of physical activity are also less frequently reported by the different black and minority ethnic communities. Again, it is Bangladeshis where the lowest rates of physical activity are reported.

Similarly, the UK population is more likely to mention dietary changes as a health-enhancing activity than any of the black and minority ethnic communities. By contrast, significant minorities of South Asians mention medical treatment in response to this question. For example, one in six older Indian and Pakistani women and over one in four older Bangladeshi women mention medication. This compares to a UK average of 4%.

Table 28: Types of health-enhancing activity engaged in (Source: AS Q34c; AC Q43)

| | | All | Women | | | Men | | |
| | | | 16–29 | 30–49 | 50–74 | 16–29 | 30–49 | 50–74 |
		%	%	%	%	%	%	%
Any	UK population	62	61	57	63	67	60	59
activity	African-Caribbean	55	48	59	45	65	63	48
	Indian	46	37	33	50	61	50	53
	Pakistani	41	31	30	43	62	39	44
	Bangladeshi	37	27	29	38	59	33	36
Sports-based	UK population	39	50	37	24	58	43	25
activity	African-Caribbean	30	27	33	17	42	45	12
	Indian	29	28	15	11	54	36	18
	Pakistani	24	17	10	9	55	26	11
	Bangladeshi	20	17	2	0	55	18	3
General	UK population	22	12	19	34	12	17	37
physical activity	African-Caribbean	10	9	4	9	11	7	23
	Indian	12	10	5	15	9	12	29
	Pakistani	8	9	8	14	4	8	11
	Bangladeshi	5	3	4	0	5	4	10
Diet	UK population	18	16	25	28	7	14	16
	African-Caribbean	8	9	15	9	4	7	5
	Indian	11	10	12	18	4	7	25
	Pakistani	8	9	8	1	4	7	16
	Bangladeshi	7	6	7	2	7	4	11
Medical	UK population	2	2	2	4	1	2	4
treatment	African-Caribbean	4	1	5	8	<0.5	3	12
	Indian	6	<0.5	6	17	1	9	6
	Pakistani	6	5	9	16	1	3	11
	Bangladeshi	10	4	19	27	1	5	18
Other lifestyle	UK population	2	2	3	3	2	3	3
modifications	African-Caribbean	1	2	2	1	1	1	0
	Indian	1	0	<0.5	4	1	1	1
	Pakistani	1	0	1	0	<0.5	1	1
	Bangladeshi	1	0	1	0	2	1	3

Base: All adults

4. Use of health services

Registration with a GP

Table 29a shows that registration with a general practitioner is almost universal. Both the UK-wide Health and Lifestyles Survey, and the current surveys amongst African-Caribbeans and South Asians found that only extremely small proportions do not report to be registered with a GP. The incidence of non-registration appears to be slightly higher amongst African-Caribbean men (4%).

This survey also shows that private medical cover for primary health care services is very limited (Table 29b). The UK figure for private medical cover for primary care services is 3%. African-Caribbeans report the same extent of cover, whilst South Asians report lower rates.

Table 29a: Extent of registration with GP (Source: AS Q46; AC Q66)

Demographic group	All adults				UK population %
	African-Caribbean %	Indian %	Pakistani %	Bangladeshi %	
All	98	100	100	100	99
Women	100	100	100	100	99
16–29	100	100	100	100	98
30–49	99	100	100	100	100
50–74	100	100	100	100	100
Men	96	100	99	100	99
16–29	97	100	98	100	97
30–49	94	100	100	100	99
50–74	99	100	100	100	100

Base: All adults

Table 29b: Private medical cover (Source: AS Q47; AC Q67)

Demographic group	All adults				UK population %
	African-Caribbean %	Indian %	Pakistani %	Bangladeshi %	
All	3	1	1	<0.5	3
Women	2	1	<0.5	0	2
16–29	4	3	1	0	2
30–49	1	0	0	0	3
50–74	2	<0.5	0	0	2
Men	3	<0.5	1	<0.5	4
16–29	3	2	0	1	3
30–49	5	0	3	0	4
50–74	3	<0.5	1	0	4

Base: All adults

Use of primary care services

Previous research on service utilisation consistently highlighted differences in consultation rates between different ethnic groups. A survey in the West Midlands, carried out in the early 1980s, showed significantly higher usage of primary care services amongst Asians, and especially Asian elders (Johnson, 1986), but also reported under-usage by young Asians (Blakemore, 1983). Data from the General Household Survey (Balarajan et al., 1989) also confirms higher rates of consultation of general practitioners amongst South Asians and African-Caribbeans. These differences in usage are particularly wide amongst older age groups. Other substantial data come from the Third National Morbidity Survey of General Practices (MSGP3), which shows higher consultation rates amongst African-Caribbeans and South Asians (McCormick et al., 1990).

The only recent survey evidence which presents a contrary picture is the re-analysis of the South Asian and black data from the North West Thames Regional Health Authority's Health and Lifestyle Survey (Nzegwu, 1993). This survey focuses on GP consultation rates within a two-week period and the reported consultation rates for a two-week period were 17% for Asians, 16% for Africans (which includes African-Caribbeans), and 18% for Europeans.

The current survey shows that GP consultation is significantly higher amongst African-Caribbeans and South Asians than the UK population at large (Table 30). For example, within a one-week period, 10% of the population covered in the national Health and Lifestyles Survey report to have used their general practitioner. Amongst African-Caribbeans, the figure is 13%, and amongst South Asians it averages at 16%. Within a one-month period, the UK figure is 28%; this rises to 32% of African-Caribbeans, 36% of Indians, 44% of Pakistanis, and 45% of Bangladeshis.

Subsequently, the average number of consultations for each population group varies (Table 31). On the basis of the UK-wide Health and Lifestyles Survey, it is estimated that the average annual consultation rate per head of population is 3.6. Amongst

African-Caribbeans it is 4.2, and amongst Indians it is 5.0. The highest consultation rates are found for Pakistanis (7.1) and Bangladeshis (7.9).

All the previous evidence has suggested increases in consultation with age amongst black and minority ethnic populations. For example, whilst the General Household Survey suggests an almost constant ratio of consultation across the different ages for the white population, it shows significant increases amongst the different black and minority ethnic populations in the 45 to 64 year old age band (Balarajan et al., 1989). The same pattern was found in the survey in the West Midlands (Blakemore, 1983), and in other local surveys (e.g. Ebrahim et al., 1991; Norman, 1985).

These patterns are very much supported by the current survey. Focusing on GP consultation within a one-month period (shown at the bottom of Table 30), the UK-wide survey shows a stable usage pattern amongst women (33% of 16 to 29 year olds use their GP within a one-month period, compared to 35% of those aged 50 to 74). Amongst men, usage rates are significantly lower in the younger and middle-aged age bands, but increase to the same level as women amongst those aged 50 to 74.

Amongst African-Caribbeans, GP usage within a one-month period is broadly similar for men and women under the age of 50. However, for the 50 to 74 year old age group, usage increases sharply to 51% of women, and 43% of men.

Amongst Indian women, consultation rates for the younger and middle age bands are similar to those of the UK population at large. Older Indian women, however, show an increased consultation rate. Indian men in general show higher consultation rates than the UK population.

Very high rates of consultation can be found amongst Pakistanis. For example, within a one-month period, 57% of Pakistani women aged 30 to 49 report to have consulted their GP, and 68% of those aged 50 to 74. Consultation rates for Pakistani men also are well above the UK average, with 35% and 50% for the respective age bands.

Table 30 also shows the higher rates in the average number of consultations for a one-year period. For Pakistani women aged 30 to 49, the average annual consultation rate is 10.3, and this rises to 13.0 for those aged 50 to 74. The comparable figures for Pakistani men are 5.3 and 9.1.

Amongst Bangladeshis, the consultation rates match those of the Pakistani population. Again, high numbers of visits are reported by the older age group, with 66% of Bangladeshi women reporting to have seen their GP in the past month. Older Bangladeshi men report consultation rates in excess of those for women. Almost three-quarters (72%) report to have seen their GP in the past month, and the average number of consultations per year for this group is 15.3.

Table 30: Last visit to surgery (Source: AS Q60; AC Q86)

		All %	Women 16–29 %	Women 30–49 %	Women 50–74 %	Men 16–29 %	Men 30–49 %	Men 50–74 %
Last week	UK population	10	12	12	12	6	7	12
	African-Caribbean	13	11	15	26	2	11	17
	Indian	16	16	16	17	9	15	24
	Pakistani	17	17	22	28	10	15	17
	Bangladeshi	15	9	19	33	5	13	30
Over 1 week, within 1 month	UK population	18	21	19	23	11	13	20
	African-Caribbean	20	30	22	25	10	7	26
	Indian	20	18	19	28	16	17	28
	Pakistani	27	26	35	40	20	20	33
	Bangladeshi	30	27	32	33	22	27	42
Over 1 month, within 2 months	UK population	12	14	12	13	11	7	14
	African-Caribbean	11	11	13	18	8	7	8
	Indian	15	14	13	29	13	13	15
	Pakistani	13	14	11	15	12	9	21
	Bangladeshi	13	12	18	11	15	11	9
Over 2 months, within 6 months	UK population	21	26	23	19	23	18	20
	African-Caribbean	17	17	17	16	16	14	25
	Indian	19	22	25	16	24	16	9
	Pakistani	23	24	23	13	26	24	22
	Bangladeshi	20	31	22	18	12	20	12
Over 6 months, within 1 year	UK population	13	12	14	11	15	14	9
	African-Caribbean	13	16	12	6	17	17	7
	Indian	8	10	7	8	9	10	6
	Pakistani	6	8	4	2	8	8	2
	Bangladeshi	6	7	4	2	13	5	2
Over 1 year ago	UK population	24	12	18	20	31	36	24
	African-Caribbean	23	11	21	9	44	36	17
	Indian	21	19	19	2	29	27	18
	Pakistani	13	13	4	3	26	23	5
	Bangladeshi	15	15	5	2	30	22	4
Within 1 month (= last week + over 1 week, within 1 month)	UK population	28	33	31	35	17	20	32
	African-Caribbean	33	41	37	51	22	18	43
	Indian	36	34	35	45	25	32	52
	Pakistani	44	43	57	68	30	35	50
	Bangladeshi	45	36	51	66	27	40	72

Base: All adults

57

Table 31: Number of times visited surgery over last 12 months (Source: AS Q61; AC Q87)

			Women			Men		
		All	16–29	30–49	50–74	16–29	30–49	50–74
		%	%	%	%	%	%	%
No. of	UK population	4.9	5.9	5.0	5.6	3.6	3.6	5.4
consultations	African-Caribbean	4.2	4.7	5.0	5.8	1.5	2.6	6.1
	Indian	5.0	4.3	4.9	9.0	2.8	4.1	8.5
	Pakistani	7.1	6.8	10.3	13.0	3.0	5.3	9.1
	Bangladeshi	7.9	5.2	10.4	12.1	3.1	6.3	15.3

Base: All adults

There has been considerable discussion on the possible underlying reasons for the higher rates of service usage amongst black and minority ethnic communities. In the perception of many GPs, Asians tend to visit surgeries more frequently with 'trivial complaints' or 'ill-defined conditions' (see Wright, 1983; Gillam *et al.*, 1989) which has led some to suggest that there is a tendency to somatise complaints (Ball, 1987).

Evidence from the Third National Morbidity Survey (McCormick *et al.*, 1990) shows that the standardised patient consultation ratios for African-Caribbeans and South Asians are particularly high for serious conditions. The evidence contained in the current survey also suggests that the health profile of black and ethnic minority communities, especially of South Asians, is worse than that of the UK population.

Reason for last visit to GP

Table 32 shows the reasons participants in the survey gave for last visiting their GP. In the UK-wide survey 53% of men and 45% of women visited the surgery for treatment. Comparative figures for women from black and South Asian communities are very similar, with the exception of Pakistani women, where 59% mentioned that they last visited for treatment. Amongst men, Pakistani and Bangladeshi men are particularly likely to mention going to their GP for treatment (60% and 63% respectively).

The second most frequently mentioned reason is to collect or order a prescription. Amongst all the different black and minority ethnic communities, men are more likely to mention this, than men in the UK-wide survey.

The third most frequently cited reason is attendance for a check-up. Compared to the UK average, Pakistani and Bangladeshi men are less likely to report that they last attended for a check-up with their GP.

Table 32 shows a number of other variations between the UK-wide data, and the findings of the current surveys. For example, Bangladeshi men and women, and Pakistani men are significantly less likely to mention blood pressure checks than their white peers. Similarly, women from all of the black and minority ethnic groups are significantly less likely to mention attendance for a cervical smear than white women. This issue is discussed in more detail in the section on cancer screening.

Table 32: Reasons for visiting surgery (Source: AS Q64; AC Q92)

	Women				Men				UK population	
	African-Caribbean %	Indian %	Pakis-tani %	Bangla-deshi %	African-Caribbean %	Indian %	Pakis-tani %	Bangla-deshi %	Women %	Men %
Treatment	44	44	59	55	49	45	60	63	45	53
Collect/order prescription	14	24	15	14	20	26	20	20	19	14
Check-up	14	14	10	12	10	12	5	9	10	14
Blood pressure check	12	8	7	4	13	11	3	4	9	9
Check ongoing condition	4	10	3	10	5	9	4	12	5	5
Blood test	2	4	3	4	6	4	1	2	4	4
Vaccination	1	5	7	2	4	7	7	4	3	4
Cervical smear	3	4	3	1	0	0	0	0	7	<0.5
Sick note/certificate	4	2	2	<0.5	4	4	4	4	2	5
Antenatal clinic	3	5	4	7	0	1	0	0	3	0
Receive results of a test	1	2	3	<0.5	0	3	<0.5	0	3	3
Make appointment	1	3	2	2	2	3	2	1	1	2
Contraception advice	3	1	1	3	0	0	0	0	4	<0.5
Asthma clinic	1	<0.5	<0.5	1	3	1	2	1	1	<0.5
Referral to specialist	3	<0.5	1	<0.5	<0.5	2	1	0	1	2
Family planning clinic	2	1	1	2	0	0	0	0	3	<0.5
Other clinic	1	<0.5	0	0	0	0	0	1	2	1

Base: All visited surgery in last 12 months

Physical access to GPs

In the UK-wide survey, 5% of the population describe physical access to their surgery as difficult (Table 33). The proportions who describe access as difficult are significantly higher amongst South Asians, particularly Bangladeshis (17% describe access as difficult).

The further analysis for the other ethnic groups by age and gender shows that Pakistani women, and older Indians and African-Caribbeans also are significantly more likely to describe GP access as difficult.

Table 33: Difficulties with access to GP (Source: AS Q59; AC Q78)

Demographic group	All adults				Standardised				
	African-Caribbean %	Indian %	Pakis-tani %	Bangla-deshi %	African-Caribbean %	Indian %	Pakis-tani %	Bangla-deshi %	UK population %
All	6	9	11	17	7	9	11	17	5
Women	7	11	16	18	8	12	16	18	7
16–29	7	7	15	16	8	8	15	16	7
30–49	6	9	15	20	6	11	17	20	5
50–74	11	23	18	17	10	18	18	17	9
Men	5	7	7	17	7	7	7	16	4
16–29	2	4	6	19	4	4	4	19	5
30–49	4	5	8	12	4	6	9	13	2
50–74	10	14	9	17	10	13	10	18	5

Base: All registered with GP

In the UK-wide survey 51% of those who have access difficulties report that their surgery is too far away (Table 34). The survey does not cover the actual distance between respondents' residence and their GP's surgery. It must be remembered that car ownership is significantly lower amongst black and minority ethnic groups.

Table 34: Reasons why access to surgery difficult (Source: AS Q59; AC Q79)

	All adults				Standardised				
	African-Caribbean %	Indian %	Pakis-tani %	Bangla-deshi %	African-Caribbean %	Indian %	Pakis-tani %	Bangla-deshi %	UK population %
Surgery hours inconvenient	3	14	5	4	2	16	5	4	9
Too far away	57	62	68	74	53	65	67	74	51
Poor public transport	41	9	10	16	40	11	11	15	25
Difficult to park	0	5	2	2	0	3	2	2	8
High crime area	0	1	4	2	0	1	4	2	0
Poor access for disabled/elderly	0	1	1	0	0	2	1	0	3
Difficulty in walking	21	20	19	12	26	17	17	13	14

Base: All who find access to surgery difficult

Appointments and waiting times

Previous surveys have shown that patients from black and minority ethnic communities are significantly more likely to attend open GP surgeries (surgeries which do not operate an appointment system) than comparative white groups (Nzegwu, 1993). In addition, there is evidence that patients from black and minority ethnic communities experience longer waiting periods at the surgery before being seen by their GP (Badger *et al.*, 1982; Jain *et al.*, 1985).

The current survey supports these findings. Table 35 shows that whilst 79% of the UK population attend appointment-based surgeries, this falls to two-thirds of African-Caribbeans, and just over half of South Asians.

Table 35: Making appointments (Source: AS Q63; AC Q91)

		All	Women			Men		
			16–29	30–49	50–74	16–29	30–49	50–74
Made an appointment	UK population	79	80	79	82	76	79	77
	African-Caribbean	65	62	62	64	74	63	66
	Indian	54	49	59	61	48	51	53
	Pakistani	52	56	57	40	49	45	54
	Bangladeshi	53	54	57	65	47	56	44
Just turned up	UK population	16	15	15	12	21	17	18
	African-Caribbean	34	37	36	36	24	34	32
	Indian	44	47	37	35	47	48	47
	Pakistani	47	40	43	57	50	54	46
	Bangladeshi	46	46	39	35	53	43	55
Asked to attend	UK population	4	4	5	5	2	3	4
	African-Caribbean	1	1	1	0	2	3	1
	Indian	2	4	3	0	2	0	2
	Pakistani	1	2	2	3	1	<0.5	0
	Bangladeshi	1	1	2	0	0	0	0

Base: All visited surgery in last 12 months

Table 36 shows that the average waiting period for black and minority ethnic communities is significantly longer than that for the UK average. The average wait for the UK population, as assessed in the Health and Lifestyles Survey, is 18 minutes. For African-Caribbeans it is 27 minutes, and for Indians 30 minutes. For Pakistanis it rises to 33 minutes, and for Bangladeshis it is 50 minutes. Although some of these differences will be based on the wider use of open surgery by members of the different black and minority ethnic communities, these differences are too large to be accounted for by this factor alone.

Not surprisingly, the proportions of patients amongst black and minority ethnic communities who wait in excess of 30 minutes is significantly higher than the UK average. In the UK-wide Health and Lifestyles Survey, 11% of the population wait in excess of 30 minutes before being seen by their GP. Amongst African-Caribbeans this rises to 19%, and amongst Indians to 23%. The proportion of Pakistanis who wait more than 30 minutes is 27%. Amongst Bangladeshis exactly half wait in excess of 30 minutes.

The final set of figures at the bottom of Table 36 shows the proportion of patients who describe the waiting period as too long. As would be expected, patients from black and minority ethnic communities are much less satisfied with the amount of time they spend waiting to be seen by their GP. For the UK average, 25% describe their waiting time as too long. Around 40% of African-Caribbeans, Indians, and Pakistanis describe the waiting time at their last visit as too long. The highest dissatisfaction is found amongst Bangladeshis, where 58% describe the waiting period as too long.

Table 36: Waiting time before seeing doctor (Source: AC Q93/94; AS Q65/66)

| | | All | Women | | | Men | | |
			16–29	30–49	50–74	16–29	30–49	50–74
Average time waited (minutes)	UK population	18	20	17	15	19	18	17
	African-Caribbean	27	28	32	26	20	24	26
	Indian	30	29	28	46	22	31	26
	Pakistani	33	32	30	41	36	34	33
	Bangladeshi	50	49	52	49	49	46	52
Proportion waiting more than 30 minutes (%)	UK population	11	13	12	6	14	13	9
	African-Caribbean	19	20	27	12	15	14	19
	Indian	23	24	24	36	18	28	11
	Pakistani	27	23	19	36	34	33	25
	Bangladeshi	50	44	50	46	48	47	60
Proportion saying waiting too long (%)	UK population	25	36	27	16	27	26	17
	African-Caribbean	40	51	47	24	49	38	21
	Indian	42	44	42	51	38	41	31
	Pakistani	39	35	31	29	52	43	44
	Bangladeshi	58	58	57	46	54	60	66

Base: All those who saw doctor at last visit

Ethnicity of GP

Table 37 shows the ethnicity of GPs, as perceived by users of GP services. The UK-wide Health and Lifestyles Survey shows that 79% see a white GP, 15% describe their GP as Asian, 1% describe their GP as West Indian, and small fractions mention Chinese or African GPs.

Amongst African-Caribbeans, equal proportions see white and Asian GPs (45%). Only 3% describe their GP as West Indian or African.

For the South Asian population groups, the ethnic identity of their GP is the mirror image of that of the white population. Over four in five South Asians attend surgeries with an Asian GP, and less than one in five attend surgeries with a white GP. Even amongst the younger age groups, only around one in five South Asians describe their GP as white.

Table 37: Ethnicity of GP (Source: AS Q50; AC Q70)

Ethnicity of GP		All %	Women			Men		
			16–29 %	30–49 %	50–74 %	16–29 %	30–49 %	50–74 %
White	UK population	79	75	80	85	77	76	79
	African-Caribbean	45	43	36	40	54	58	38
	Indian	14	15	11	8	19	17	10
	Pakistani	15	18	9	9	22	16	10
	Bangladeshi	19	19	22	19	16	20	17
Asian	UK population	15	16	14	10	17	18	17
	African-Caribbean	45	46	48	52	41	36	49
	Indian	81	82	86	86	70	80	80
	Pakistani	83	80	87	91	75	82	89
	Bangladeshi	80	79	78	81	82	79	80
Chinese	UK population	<0.5	1	<0.5	<0.5	1	<0.5	<0.5
	African-Caribbean	3	4	3	3	0	2	3
	Indian	1	0	1	<0.5	5	0	1
	Pakistani	<0.5	0	0	0	<0.5	0	<0.5
	Bangladeshi	0	0	0	0	0	0	0
African	UK population	<0.5	<0.5	0	<0.5	<0.5	<0.5	<0.5
	African-Caribbean	2	2	4	1	1	0	5
	Indian	<0.5	0	0	0	0	1	0
	Pakistani	<0.5	<0.5	<0.5	0	0	0	0
	Bangladeshi	<0.5	0	0	0	0	0	<0.5
West Indian	UK population	1	1	2	1	1	1	<0.5
	African-Caribbean	1	1	1	1	<0.5	1	3
	Indian	0	0	0	0	0	0	0
	Pakistani	<0.5	0	0	0	0	0	<0.5
	Bangladeshi	0	0	0	0	0	0	0
It varies	UK population	2	3	2	3	1	3	1
	African-Caribbean	4	3	8	7	2	3	4
	Indian	3	3	1	4	4	1	9
	Pakistani	2	1	4	0	<0.5	2	1
	Bangladeshi	1	3	0	0	1	1	0

Base: All registered with GP

Language of communication

Chapter 2 shows that high proportions of the South Asian communities do not consider English as their main language. All those who do not describe English as their main language were asked how they communicate with their GP (Table 38).

Amongst Indians who do not describe English as their main language, 59% communicate in one of the Asian languages, and 41% in English. Women are more likely to communicate with their GP in one of the South Asian languages than men, and use of mother tongue or another South Asian language increases across age bands. Amongst Pakistanis and Bangladeshis who do not describe their main language as English, the proportion who rely on English as their means of communicating with their GP is around 35%. The remaining two-thirds communicate in one of the South Asian languages. For both groups the gender and age pattern found amongst Indians is repeated. Small proportions of South Asians communicate in more than one language. It seems likely that this occurs in practices with more than one GP.

The figures reported in Table 38 are based on all those who do not describe English as their main language. For the population groups as a whole, one can therefore estimate that 40% of Indians communicate with their GP in one of the South Asian languages; amongst Pakistanis 50% communicate in their mother tongue or another South Asian language, and amongst Bangladeshis 59% do so.

Table 38: Language of communication with GP (Source: AS Q51)

Ethnic group	Language of communication	All %	Women 16–29 %	Women 30–49 %	Women 50–74 %	Men 16–29 %	Men 30–49 %	Men 50–74 %
Indians	English	41	50	38	19	67	49	35
	Gujerati	23	20	27	23	16	22	20
	Punjabi	22	13	23	29	13	19	31
	Hindi	21	20	20	27	16	20	20
	Urdu	8	17	6	3	3	9	9
Pakistani	Urdu	42	30	47	43	27	51	43
	English	34	48	20	10	67	41	30
	Punjabi	30	27	29	45	18	24	39
Bangladeshi	Bengali	47	39	53	54	34	55	52
	English	35	39	19	8	71	33	27
	Sylheti	8	10	11	13	3	9	6
	Urdu	7	2	5	3	1	8	19

Base: All those whose main language is not English

Use of interpreters

Table 39 shows the extent to which South Asians, who do not describe English as their main language, make use of formal or informal interpreters. Amongst Indians, 4% have on occasion used informal interpreters, and 3% report that their GP surgery has on occasion provided interpreting services. Amongst Pakistanis, 4% report to have used informal interpreters and 1% say their GP practice has on occasion provided interpreting services.

Not surprisingly, the highest proportion who report the use of informal interpreters is found amongst Bangladeshis (12%). A further 7% report that their practice on occasion provides interpreting services.

Generally, the use of formal and informal interpreting increases across age bands, and is significantly higher amongst women. Informal interpreting often relies on the help of the spouse, or of the son or daughter of the patient. Other research has shown that the use of informal interpreters can be problematic (CELFHSA/MORI, 1993; East London and City Health Authority/MORI, 1994). For example, the East London Survey showed that over a third of patients who use informal interpreters report difficulties. These include inhibitions in talking about women's health issues via the husband or son or daughter, as well as problems with the accuracy of interpretation.

Table 39: Use of interpreters (Source: AS Q53-56)

Ethnic group		All %	Women 16–29 %	Women 30–49 %	Women 50–74 %	Men 16–29 %	Men 30–49 %	Men 50–74 %
Indians	Use informal interpreter	4	<0.5	3	14	2	4	0
	– spouse	1	<0.5	2	<0.5	0	1	0
	– child	3	0	0	13	0	3	0
	– other	<0.5	0	1	1	2	0	0
	Interpreter provided	3	2	1	15	0	0	1
Pakistanis	Use informal interpreter	4	2	8	9	2	1	1
	– spouse	3	2	6	3	2	1	0
	– child	2	0	3	6	0	<0.5	1
	– other	<0.5	0	<0.5	0	0	0	0
	Interpreter provided	1	1	2	2	0	<0.5	1
Bangladeshis	Use informal interpreter	12	10	25	30	3	2	6
	– spouse	7	9	17	12	3	1	0
	– child	4	0	8	16	0	6	0
	– other	2	<0.5	4	12	0	0	0
	Interpreter provided	7	8	12	16	3	2	7

Base: All those whose main language is not English

Almost all South Asians feel that it is very or fairly easy to understand their GP (Table 40). Amongst Indians and Pakistanis, 2% and 3% respectively do not feel that it is easy to understand their GP, and amongst Bangladeshis the figure rises to 8%.

Difficulties are more pronounced amongst Bangladeshi women aged 30 to 49, where 16% do not feel it is easy to communicate with their GP, and amongst women aged 50 to 74, where 14% fall into this category. Similarly, amongst older Bangladeshi men, 12% feel it is not easy to understand their GP.

Table 40: Very/fairly easy to understand GP/doctor (Source: AS Q52; AC Q72)

Demographic group	All adults		
	Indian	Pakistani	Bangladeshi
All	98	97	92
Women	97	97	88
16-29	99	98	92
30-49	98	95	84
50-74	96	98	86
Men	98	98	94
16-29	100	94	99
30-49	97	99	98
50-74	99	99	88

Base: Those whose main language is not English

Quality of communication

The survey explores in further detail the quality of the interaction between GPs and users from the various black and minority ethnic communities. The first set of findings in Table 41 shows the proportion of GP users who feel they were given a full explanation about their condition or treatment at their last visit. Bangladeshi GP users are most likely to agree that they have been given a full explanation about their condition and treatment.

The second set of findings in Table 41 shows that almost all recent users who have been given an explanation about their treatment or condition feel that this was easy to understand. As we have already shown in Table 40, amongst Bangladeshis, sizeable minorities (12%) experienced some difficulties in understanding the explanation offered by their GP. However, less than half of those with difficulties feel that this is due to language problems.

Table 41: Quality of communication with GP (Source: AS Q67; AC Q97)

		All	Women			Men		
			16–29	30–49	50–74	16–29	30–49	50–74
		%	%	%	%	%	%	%
Proportion who felt they were given an explanation	UK population	73	69	78	67	78	78	71
	African-Caribbean	67	62	76	62	70	61	70
	Indian	69	64	77	73	59	64	78
	Pakistani	69	62	76	75	60	72	73
	Bangladeshi	81	86	85	85	63	81	90

Base: All visited doctor

		All	Women			Men		
Proportion who felt the explanation was easy to understand	UK population	97	94	96	99	96	97	98
	African-Caribbean	98	94	99	97	100	100	99
	Indian	97	92	97	100	99	98	95
	Pakistani	99	99	100	100	95	100	98
	Bangladeshi	88	97	80	91	87	94	82
Proportion who felt the explanation was difficult due to language problems	Indian	1	4	0	0	0	0	0
	Pakistani	<0.5	1	0	0	0	0	1
	Bangladeshi	5	1	8	3	0	3	12

Base: All given explanation

Table 42 explores other quality issues in the consultation process. The first set of data shows to what extent users of GP services feel that the amount of time their GP has spent with them during the last consultation was sufficient. In the UK-wide survey, 87% report that the time spent with their GP was sufficient; there is no gender difference, and satisfaction increases with age.

Amongst African-Caribbeans, the proportion who feel the time spent was adequate is somewhat lower at 78%. Fewer South Asians feel that the amount of time their GP spent with them was sufficient (73% of Indians and Pakistanis and 68% of Bangladeshis).

Four in five GP users across all the different ethnic groups feel that their GP was caring about their conditional problem at the last consultation. Again, it is younger users who are slightly less positive.

The third set of findings in Table 42 shows that there is some difference in the proportion of patients who feel happy with the outcome of their last visit. In the UK-wide survey, 88% feel happy with the outcome of their most recent visit. Amongst African-Caribbeans, the respective figure is 83%. Amongst South Asians figures tend to be somewhat lower; 81% of Pakistanis report satisfaction with their most recent visit, as do 78% of Indians. The lowest satisfaction rating is found amongst Bangladeshis (72%).

Table 42: Quality of consultation (Source: AS Q67; AC Q97)

		All	Women			Men		
			16–29	30–49	50–74	16–29	30–49	50–74
		%	%	%	%	%	%	%
Proportion saying time spent with doctor was long enough	UK population	87	79	89	91	81	87	91
	African-Caribbean	78	70	82	85	76	68	90
	Indian	73	70	76	84	60	69	79
	Pakistani	73	72	73	74	64	79	76
	Bangladeshi	68	65	67	72	67	68	75
Proportion who felt GP cared about condition/problem	UK population	81	72	86	86	74	78	87
	African-Caribbean	76	63	81	81	79	73	87
	Indian	81	67	83	91	69	86	91
	Pakistani	82	74	92	83	69	88	88
	Bangladeshi	82	80	86	80	73	79	91
Proportion who were happy with outcome of the visit	UK population	88	83	89	89	87	88	92
	African-Caribbean	83	77	85	92	83	65	94
	Indian	78	71	79	91	68	78	87
	Pakistani	81	81	83	80	71	86	83
	Bangladeshi	72	70	70	56	70	75	81

Base: All who visited doctor

Gender preference for GP

Table 43 shows to what extent members of the different communities have access to GPs of their own gender, and what the gender preference for their GP is. The issue of greatest interest here is to what extent women are currently seeing female GPs, and how strong their preference for seeing a female GP is.

At present between three-quarters and four-fifths of men see male GPs. Amongst women on average less than one in five see female GPs. However, there is a significant number of women who currently see a male GP or who attend practices where they see both male and female GPs, who actually prefer to see female GPs.

In the UK-wide survey, 18% of women are currently seeing a female GP. An additional 10% currently see a male GP but prefer to see a female GP, and a further 4% currently see both male and female GPs but prefer to see a female GP.

For African-Caribbean women broadly similar figures are shown in Table 43.

Preferences for a female GP are much stronger amongst South Asian women. When combining those who currently see a male GP and those who see both male and female GPs, an additional 30% prefer to see female GPs (above the 20% who already see a female GP). Amongst young Pakistani women, an additional 38% prefer to see a female GP and amongst Bangladeshi women an additional 41% have a preference for a female GP.

Preference for a female GP rises slightly amongst the 30 to 49 year old age group, and falls back slightly amongst those aged 50 to 74.

These figures demonstrate that for South Asian women, especially those of Pakistani and Bangladeshi origin, access to a female GP is preferred.

Table 43: Gender preference for GP (Source: AS Q48/49; AC Q68/69)

| | | All | Women | | | Men | | |
| | | | 16–29 | 30–49 | 50–74 | 16–29 | 30–49 | 50–74 |
		%	%	%	%	%	%	%
Currently see same-sex GP	UK population	47	19	17	16	76	75	81
	African-Caribbean	42	27	24	15	69	65	82
	Indian	44	20	13	10	77	76	75
	Pakistani	50	20	14	25	81	83	86
	Bangladeshi	50	22	18	21	84	83	79
Currently see opposite-sex GP, but prefer same-sex GP	UK population	5	12	10	7	<0.5	<0.5	1
	African-Caribbean	6	14	5	8	0	3	0
	Indian	15	25	30	19	1	4	2
	Pakistani	17	33	34	25	3	1	1
	Bangladeshi	17	34	34	26	2	1	0
Currently see male and female GP, but prefer same-sex GP	UK population	3	4	4	3	2	1	2
	African-Caribbean	2	3	6	2	0	0	1
	Indian	4	5	7	5	3	2	2
	Pakistani	5	5	10	5	2	1	2
	Bangladeshi	8	8	10	14	4	7	5

Base: All adults registered with GP

Contact with other members of the primary care team

The survey also assessed the extent to which black and minority ethnic communities have access to other members of the primary care team. The UK-wide Health and Lifestyles Survey shows that the key contact is with general practitioners (85%). Table 44 shows that high proportions also came into contact with the practice receptionist during their last visit (71%). However, there is much more limited contact with any other member of the primary care team. The only professional group mentioned frequently are practice nurses (20%).

The comparative data for African-Caribbeans and South Asians show that there is a significantly stronger dependence on GPs, and generally lower rates of contact with any other member of the primary care team. This is particularly the case for men from the South Asian communities.

The greatest dependence on the general practitioner can be found amongst Bangladeshis. Here, 98% of women and 99% of men report to have seen their general practitioner during their last visit. Only 7% of Bangladeshi women (compared to 20% of the UK average) mentioned seeing their practice nurse; amongst Bangladeshi men this figure is 5%.

An additional question asked about which language users and practice nurses communicated in. Only around one in ten of those who have come into contact with a practice nurse report that they were able to communicate in their mother tongue or another South Asian language.

Table 44: Staff dealt with at last visit to surgery (Source: AS Q62; AC Q90)

	Women				Men				UK population	
	African-Caribbean	Indian	Pakis-tani	Bangla-deshi	African-Caribbean	Indian	Pakis-tani	Bangla-deshi	Women	Men
	%	%	%	%	%	%	%	%	%	%
Doctor/GP	92	94	98	98	92	94	97	99	85	84
Receptionist	76	57	62	57	57	56	70	65	71	68
Practice nurse	14	14	9	7	14	10	6	5	20	20
Practice pharmacist	2	<0.5	4	<0.5	1	2	5	<0.5	3	2
Midwife	2	3	3	2	0	<0.5	0	0	2	0
Health visitor	1	2	1	2	1	1	1	0	1	<0.5
Physio-therapist	1	<0.5	1	0	2	<0.5	<0.5	<0.5	<0.5	1

Base: All who visited surgery in last 12 months

Use of other health services

Table 45 shows the proportion of the different community groups who have used other health services. The national figures for using dental services in a 12-month period are 61% of women and 52% of men (this question was not included in the UK-wide Health and Lifestyles Survey, and the data are taken from another UK-wide survey conducted by MORI for the National Consumer Council (1993)). Broadly speaking, the rates of using dentists amongst African-Caribbeans are around 80% of those of the white population; those amongst Indians and Pakistanis are around 70% of the white population, and those amongst Bangladeshis are about half of those found in the UK population at large.

Use of opticians also varies with ethnicity. Thus, South Asian women, especially Bangladeshi women are significantly less likely to have visited an optician in the past 12 months than white women. Amongst men, African-Caribbean and Bangladeshi men are least likely to have used opticians.

Amongst women in the UK-wide survey, 12% report to have used family planning clinics in the past 12 months. Amongst South Asian women, the proportions are very similar, and amongst Bangladeshi women usage is slightly above the national average (16%). Reported use of family planning clinics is also somewhat above the national average amongst African-Caribbean women (17%).

In the UK-wide sample, 11% of women have used a health visitor in the last 12 months, and 5% have used a community midwife. The proportion of women amongst the different black and ethnic minority groups who have used either of these two services is very similar, with the exception of Indian women who report lower usage of both health visiting and community midwifery services.

Chiropodist services are used by 9% of women and 4% of men in the UK-wide sample. Usage of chiropodist services is extremely low amongst South Asians, with less than 2% of Indians, and almost none of the Pakistanis and Bangladeshis reporting to have used chiropodist services in the past 12 months.

There has been intermittent speculation by health service providers about the impact of traditional healers (hakims/vaids). Local surveys, such as the West Midlands study (Johnson, 1986) and the work by Bhopal (1986) in Glasgow, have shown that very little use is made of such traditional healers. The last set of figures in Table 45 shows the proportion of South Asians who report to have used traditional healers in the current survey. Again, this confirms that their role in health service provision is very limited.

Table 45: Services used in past year (Source: AS Q111; AC Q153)

	Women				Men				UK population	
	African-Caribbean	Indian	Pakis-tani	Bangla-deshi	African-Caribbean	Indian	Pakis-tani	Bangla-deshi	Women	Men
	%	%	%	%	%	%	%	%	%	%
Dentist	53	37	44	26	41	39	39	26	61*	52*
Optician	27	24	22	18	17	24	24	19	31	25
Family planning clinic	17	11	11	16	1	3	3	3	12	1
Health visitor	11	7	10	13	2	1	4	3	11	2
Community midwife	3	2	5	8	1	0	2	0	5	1
Chiropodist	5	1	1	0	3	2	0	0	9	4
District nurse	2	2	2	2	0	1	1	1	4	3
Hakims/vaids	NA	0	1	1	NA	0	2	0	NA	NA

Base: All adults
*not included in Health and Lifestyles Survey
Data drawn from national survey for National Consumer Council (1993)

Cancer screening

Previous studies (McAvoy and Raza, 1988; Donaldson, 1984; Balarajan and Bulusu, 1990) have all confirmed lower uptake amongst South Asians and African-Caribbean women for cancer screening programmes than amongst white women.

The current survey explored in greater detail the extent to which different groups have used cancer screening programmes. Less than 1% of any of the samples covered, including the UK-wide Health and Lifestyles Survey sample, mentioned having been screened for cancers such as skin cancer, testicular cancer, and lung cancer. Only breast cancer screening and cervical cancer screening are mentioned by large proportions of women (see Table 46).

In the UK-wide sample of 16 to 74 year old women, 60% report to ever have been screened for cancer of the cervix. Amongst African-Caribbean women the figure is 54%. The proportion of women from the different South Asian groups who report to have participated in cervical screening is significantly lower; amongst Indian women it is 37%, amongst Pakistani women 32%, and amongst Bangladeshi women 28%.

It should be noted however, that these responses are in reply to the question 'Have you ever had any screening for any type of cancer?' Table 47 shows responses to the question 'Have you ever had a cervical smear test?' which elicited a significantly higher number of positive replies. For example, 85% of the women participating in the UK-wide survey report to have had a cervical smear test, and the lowest rate is reported amongst Bangladeshi women, with 40%. This indicates that amongst all groups of women, high proportions are not aware of the purpose of cervical screening.

Table 46 also shows the reported figures for breast cancer screening. Again, it seems likely that these figures are underestimates. However, there is a significant difference in reported uptake of breast cancer screening between the different ethnic groups, with the women in the UK-wide survey showing the highest uptake (21%), and Bangladeshi women reporting the lowest uptake (4%).

Table 46: Cancer screening (Source: AS Q117; AC Q159)

			Women		
		All %	16–29 %	30–49 %	50–74 %
Cervical smear	UK population	60	48	73	56
	African-Caribbean	54	45	57	63
	Indian	37	25	51	27
	Pakistani	32	23	44	28
	Bangladeshi	28	23	38	18
Breast cancer	UK population	21	3	16	41
	African-Caribbean	14	5	12	31
	Indian	7	6	5	14
	Pakistani	7	3	8	18
	Bangladeshi	4	1	5	14

Base: All women

Table 47 shows the reported incidence of cervical screening. Responses are based on a direct question asking whether women have had a cervical smear test, and are therefore likely to be more accurate than those reported in, say, Table 46. The recently published report on the *First Five Years of the NHS Cervical Screening Programme* (National Co-ordinating Network, 1994) estimates that 83% of women aged 20 to 64 in England have had a smear test in the past 5½ years. The figures found in the UK-wide Health and Lifestyles Survey show that 77% of women have had a smear test in the past five years, and a further 8% had a smear test longer ago than five years. Even when allowing for the slightly different age bands covered in the survey, these figures are reassuringly close to the statistics from the National Cervical Screening Programme.

Table 47 shows that there are significant differences between African-Caribbeans and South Asian women. Whilst uptake amongst African-Caribbean women is very similar to the UK average (81% report to have had a test in the last 5 years, and a further 6% longer ago than 5 years), the figures for women from the South Asian communities are significantly lower. Amongst Indian women, 63% report to have had a smear test in the past 5 years, and a further 3% longer ago than that. Amongst Pakistani women less than half (45%) have had a test in the past five years, and amongst Bangladeshi women this figure falls to 33%.

Uptake is particularly low in the youngest and oldest age bands of South Asian women. For example, amongst younger Indian women, 43% report never to have had a smear test; amongst the older group this figure is 38%.

Table 47: Cervical smear (Source: AS Q119; AC Q161)

		All %	Women 16–29 %	30–49 %	50–74 %
In last 6 months	UK population	15	18	19	9
	African-Caribbean	17	23	17	5
	Indian	16	14	22	6
	Pakistani	10	9	11	12
	Bangladeshi	7	6	8	5
Over 6 months within 12 months	UK population	15	17	20	8
	African-Caribbean	19	21	17	17
	Indian	14	15	16	8
	Pakistani	10	9	11	9
	Bangladeshi	5	7	5	1
Over 1 year within 3 years	UK population	34	30	42	30
	African-Caribbean	35	28	41	36
	Indian	26	21	31	23
	Pakistani	21	16	29	13
	Bangladeshi	16	13	21	14
Over 3 years within 5 years	UK population	10	6	10	13
	African-Caribbean	8	4	10	13
	Indian	7	4	6	13
	Pakistani	4	3	7	2
	Bangladeshi	5	1	10	0
Over 5 years	UK population	8	1	4	19
	African-Caribbean	6	1	8	11
	Indian	3	2	3	4
	Pakistani	4	0	9	4
	Bangladeshi	1	0	1	1
Never	UK population	15	29	3	18
	African-Caribbean	13	23	2	13
	Indian	30	43	17	38
	Pakistani	46	62	31	36
	Bangladeshi	60	70	43	71

Base: All women

Table 48 shows that there are significant differences in the proportion of women who report to have been encouraged by a health professional to have a cervical smear test. In the UK-wide survey, 36% of women report to have received encouragement from a health professional in the last 12 months. Amongst African-Caribbean and Indian women slightly higher proportions report to have had such encouragement (39% and 43% respectively). Pakistani and Bangladeshi women are significantly less likely to report having received such encouragement in the past 12 months (25% and 22% respectively).

Table 48: Health professional suggested having smear test in last 12 months (Source: AS Q120; AC Q162)

| Demographic group | All women | | | | UK population |
	African-Caribbean %	Indian %	Pakistani %	Bangla-deshi %	Women %
All	39	43	25	22	36
Women					
16–29	48	38	25	20	40
30–49	34	52	26	23	41
50–74	31	32	23	21	28

Base: All women

Amongst women in the UK-wide sample, the main reason for not having a cervical smear test was that the woman did not feel the need to have such a test (28%), followed closely by the lack of encouragement or information provided (24%). A sizeable proportion of women say that they have been too busy to have the test (this is a particularly important reason for women aged 30 to 49), or report that they do not feel they need to be screened since they are not sexually active (11%).

The reasons for not having a smear test given by women from the different black and ethnic minority communities are shown in Table 49. For African-Caribbean women, the most frequently mentioned reasons are that women do not feel the need for it (37%) or have not been sexually active (19%). Smaller proportions mention that they have not been informed about the test (11%) or have been too busy (10%).

For South Asian women information appears to be a critical factor. Whilst hardly any of the women in the UK-wide survey, or African-Caribbean women report that they do not know what a smear test is, sizeable proportions of South Asian women appear to lack information. When combining the proportions who report never to have been given an appointment for a test and those who report not to know what the test is, 35% of Indian women who have not been screened appear to lack basic information about cervical screening. Amongst Pakistani women who have not been screened this proportion rises to 48%, and amongst Bangladeshi non-attenders to 52%.

The data contained in Table 49, and the information shown previously about the lower rates of promotion of cervical screening reported by South Asian women, highlight an important information deficit.

Table 49: Reasons for not having a smear test
(Source: AS Q121; AC Q165)

		%
Don't feel I need to	UK population	28
	African-Caribbean	37
	Indian	16
	Pakistani	13
	Bangladeshi	12
Never been told/recommended to	UK population	24
	African-Caribbean	11
	Indian	22
	Pakistani	33
	Bangladeshi	18
Don't know what smear test is	UK population	1
	African-Caribbean	1
	Indian	13
	Pakistani	15
	Bangladeshi	34
Too busy/never got round to it	UK population	13
	African-Caribbean	10
	Indian	11
	Pakistani	2
	Bangladeshi	6
Never been sexually active	UK population	11
	African-Caribbean	19
	Indian	6
	Pakistani	7
	Bangladeshi	6
Embarrassment	UK population	5
	African-Caribbean	1
	Indian	5
	Pakistani	5
	Bangladeshi	3
Scared	UK population	5
	African-Caribbean	2
	Indian	5
	Pakistani	2
	Bangladeshi	<0.5

Base: All women who have never had a smear test

5. Smoking

Smoking prevalence

Existing evidence on smoking rates amongst black and minority ethnic communities is patchy, and somewhat contradictory. National estimates were derived from an analysis of the smoking prevalence data collected in the 1978 and 1980 General Household Surveys (Balarajan and Yuen, 1986). This showed that the smoking rate amongst Asians was over two-and-a-half times lower, and that of African-Caribbeans two times lower than that of the English population, after adjustment by age and gender.

Local surveys showed varying smoking prevalence rates. For example, a survey of Asians in Brent and Harrow (McKeigue *et al.*, 1985) found that amongst this group, 34% of men were current smokers; the figure for women was 1%. This group consisted mainly of Indians and East African Asians. A survey conducted amongst Bangladeshis in East London (McKeigue *et al.*, 1988) found that the smoking rates for this group (which was aged 35–69 years) were 82% for men, and 22% for women. By contrast, a survey of Asians in Ealing, who are mainly Sikh, found that 9% either currently or in the past had smoked 16 cigarettes a day or more (McKeigue *et al.*, 1993).

Another local survey, carried out amongst Asian factory workers in Bradford, found that 46% of male Muslims were current cigarette smokers and 23% of Hindus (Knight *et al.*, 1993).

These local studies show that for Asian men smoking may be a considerable risk factor. One possible reason why the analysis of the General Household Survey suggested much lower prevalence rates may be that the survey was conducted in English only. As we have shown in Chapter 1, bilingual interviewing is critical for reaching significant sections of the different Asian communities. All of the local surveys referred to above, included mother-tongue interviewing, as well as interviewing in English. Furthermore, the General Household Survey analysis groups together the different South Asian groups. As the local surveys show, smoking rates vary considerably between the different South Asian communities.

The current survey therefore combines not only the most appropriate interviewing approach but, with its wider coverage and larger sample sizes, offers more reliable insights into smoking amongst black and minority ethnic communities. Table 50 shows the proportion for each of the target communities who smoke cigarettes regularly. As in previous sections, the table shows the figures for each community group, and standardised figures for which each group's data have been weighted to the UK age and sex profile.

The UK figure for regular cigarette smoking is 28%. Amongst the different Asian groups, Bangladeshis show the highest smoking prevalence with 23%. This falls to 15% of Pakistanis, and to 10% of Indians. African-Caribbeans' smoking prevalence rate is 22%. Whilst these figures suggest that smoking is less of a risk factor for black and South Asian communities overall, the analysis by gender shows a different picture.

Amongst South Asian women, smoking rates are very low. The one group which reports slightly higher rates of smoking are Bangladeshi women aged 50 to 74. Overall, African-Caribbean women also record smoking rates below the national figure. However, amongst young African-Caribbean women smoking rates are almost identical to the comparative UK figure.

Smoking prevalence figures for men show that smoking is a considerable risk factor. Figures for African-Caribbean men and for Pakistani men are very similar to the UK figure. Indian men show the lowest smoking prevalence, but amongst Bangladeshis a significantly higher rate of smoking is recorded.

Smoking rates amongst Bangladeshi men are particularly high amongst those aged 30 to 49 (46%), and over half (56%) of those aged 50 to 74 are regular cigarette smokers. This is over twice the figure of the comparable UK age group.

For African-Caribbean men, the lowest smoking rates are found in the youngest age group; these are significantly lower than those of the matching UK figure. By contrast, older African-Caribbean men exceed the matching UK average.

Table 50: Current regular smokers % (Source: AC Q167-169/177; AS Q122-124/132)

Demographic group	All adults				Standardised				UK population %
	African-Caribbean %	Indian %	Pakis-tani %	Bangla-deshi %	African-Caribbean %	Indian %	Pakis-tani %	Bangla-deshi %	
All	22	10	15	23	22	10	16	22	28
Women	18	1	2	4	17	1	2	5	27
16–29	28	1	2	1	30	1	2	2	31
30–49	16	1	1	5	17	1	2	4	29
50–74	3	1	2	12	5	2	2	12	21
Men	28	19	28	40	29	20	30	42	29
16–29	23	19	23	26	22	20	26	28	30
30–49	28	21	36	44	29	20	38	46	31
50–74	33	17	20	57	33	21	23	56	25

Base: All adults

Table 51 shows the proportions of each demographic group who have ever smoked either a cigarette, cigar or pipe. Figures show that the majority of the UK population (73%) have at least experimented with smoking at some stage in their lives. The same is true for over half (58%) of African-Caribbeans, but only for minorities of the South Asian community. The overall patterns by age and gender are very similar to those reported in Table 50.

Table 51: Those who have ever smoked a cigarette, cigar or pipe %
(Source: AS Q122; AC Q167)

Demographic group	All adults				Standardised				UK population
	African-Caribbean %	Indian %	Pakis-tani %	Bangla-deshi %	African-Caribbean %	Indian %	Pakis-tani %	Bangla-deshi %	%
All	58	24	29	44	55	22	29	32	73
Women	44	6	7	7	42	5	7	7	67
16–29	60	7	9	6	63	6	8	7	63
30–49	42	4	4	5	41	4	5	5	69
50–74	22	7	9	13	24	4	11	13	68
Men	74	42	49	58	73	42	51	59	78
16–29	68	42	42	45	67	41	47	46	67
30–49	79	45	51	60	79	43	53	60	78
50–74	75	35	59	74	74	39	54	74	67

Base: All adults

The questionnaire also tried to establish at what age people first experimented with smoking (Table 52), and at what age they started to smoke regularly (Table 53). These figures show that regular cigarette smokers amongst black and South Asian men started their experimentation with smoking slightly later than the average UK smoker, and that their progression to regular smoking also lagged behind by a similar interval. The number of South Asian women smokers is too small to allow further analysis.

Table 52: Average age when first tried smoking (Source: AC Q178; AS Q133)

Demographic group	All adults				Standardised				UK population
	African-Caribbean %	Indian %	Pakis-tani %	Bangla-deshi %	African-Caribbean %	Indian %	Pakis-tani %	Bangla-deshi %	%
All	16	17	16	16	16	17	16	16	15
Women	16	*	*	*	16	*	*	*	16
Men	15	16	16	16	16	16	16	16	14

Base: All current regular smokers
*Bases too small for breakdown

Table 53: Average age when started to smoke regularly (Source: AC Q179; AS Q134)

Demographic group	All adults				Standardised				UK population
	African-Caribbean %	Indian %	Pakis-tani %	Bangla-deshi %	African-Caribbean %	Indian %	Pakis-tani %	Bangla-deshi %	%
All	19	20	19	18	19	20	19	18	18
Women	19	*	*	*	19	*	*	*	19
Men	19	19	19	18	19	19	19	18	17

Base: All current regular smokers
*Bases too small for breakdown

Cigarette consumption

Those who report to have smoked the day prior to the interview were asked how many cigarettes they had consumed. Table 54 shows that typical daily consumption is significantly lower amongst all black and minority ethnic community groups, compared to the UK average. This is the case for both men and women, although the low number of South Asian women smokers makes any further analysis impossible.

Amongst male smokers, 22% in the UK-wide Health and Lifestyles Survey are heavy smokers (over 20 cigarettes on a typical day). Just under half (48%) smoke between 11 and 20 cigarettes (moderate smokers), and 30% smoke 10 cigarettes or less (light smokers).

The proportion of light smokers amongst black and ethnic minority men is significantly higher; for example, 68% of African-Caribbean male smokers smoke 10 or fewer cigarettes in a typical day.

Heavy smoking occurs relatively infrequently amongst African-Caribbean and South Asian male smokers. The highest rate is found for African-Caribbeans (13%), and the lowest amongst Indian men (6%).

Table 54: Average number of cigarettes smoked yesterday
(Source: AC Q182; AS Q137)

Demographic group	All adults				Standardised				UK population
	African-Caribbean %	Indian %	Pakis-tani %	Bangla-deshi %	African-Caribbean %	Indian %	Pakis-tani %	Bangla-deshi %	%
All adults									
Average number	11 cigs	11 cigs	13 cigs	11 cigs	11 cigs	11 cigs	13 cigs	11 cigs	17 cigs
Up to 5	26	19	20	23	36	28	24	29	10
6–10	46	46	30	43	38	41	30	40	22
11–15	11	17	16	13	10	15	16	12	21
16–20	9	14	26	14	8	12	23	13	28
21 or more	8	5	8	7	7	4	7	6	19
Women									
Average number	9 cigs	*	*	*	9 cigs	*	*	*	15 cigs
Up to 5	31	*	*	*	39	*	*	*	12
6–10	46	*	*	*	37	*	*	*	23
11–15	11	*	*	*	8	*	*	*	22
16–20	9	*	*	*	9	*	*	*	29
21 or more	2	*	*	*	6	*	*	*	14
Men									
Average number	12 cigs	12 cigs	13 cigs	12 cigs	13 cigs	11 cigs	13 cigs	11 cigs	18 cigs
Up to 5	22	18	20	21	33	21	23	26	8
6–10	46	46	30	44	38	43	31	41	22
11–15	10	18	17	13	8	20	16	12	21
16–20	9	14	25	15	10	12	22	15	27
21 or more	13	6	9	8	12	4	7	7	22

Base: Those who smoked yesterday
*Bases too small for breakdown

Chewing of paan, betel nut, and other substances

The preliminary qualitative research suggested that it was not uncommon for South Asians to add tobacco to a variety of chewing substances, most commonly paan. Paan is a green leaf, and is chewed with a paste made of limestone and betel nuts, which sometimes also includes coconuts or cloves. It is taken regularly, usually after meals, but some people are reported to be chewing more or less continuously.

Table 55 shows that chewing is very widespread amongst Bangladeshis (66%); but is fairly infrequent amongst Indians (15%), and Pakistanis (7%). Chewing is most widespread amongst middle-aged and older Bangladeshis. Amongst Bangladeshi women, 88% of 30 to 49 year olds report to be chewing, and amongst 50 to 74 year olds, this rises to 96%. Amongst men of the same age bands, roughly three-quarters chew.

Paan is the most commonly mentioned ingredient, with 50% of Bangladeshis reporting to be chewing paan. Consumption increases greatly with age, from 31% of younger women to 76% of older women; amongst men the increase is from 40% to 62% respectively.

It is not uncommon to add tobacco to the chewing mixture. The third set of findings in Table 55 shows that as many as 28% of Bangladeshis add tobacco to the chewing substance. This rises to 48% of Bangladeshi women aged 30 to 49, and to 58% of women aged 50 to 74. The survey did not establish the amounts chewed. The intention was, at this stage, to assess how widespread tobacco chewing was. Clearly, amongst Bangladeshi women, and to a lesser extent Bangladeshi men, the addition of tobacco to the chewing mixture is very common.

There are some local projects exploring the health risks of chewing – for example the Betel Nut project in East London (London Royal Trust, personal communication). The current survey supports the need for a more extensive investigation into the actual amounts of tobacco chewed.

Table 55: Chewing tobacco products – used nowadays (Source: AS Q154)

		All %	Women 16–29 %	Women 30–49 %	Women 50–74 %	Men 16–29 %	Men 30–49 %	Men 50–74 %
Any chewing product	Indian	15	6	12	17	10	23	23
	Pakistani	7	7	10	8	4	7	11
	Bangladeshi	66	43	88	96	49	76	74
Paan	Indian	10	5	8	11	8	16	16
	Pakistani	4	5	6	1	2	5	5
	Bangladeshi	50	31	59	76	40	58	62
Any tobacco product	Indian	4	2	3	4	1	3	12
	Pakistani	1	1	1	2	1	1	2
	Bangladeshi	28	14	48	58	13	31	31
Betel nut/ sopari chewed with tobacco	Indian	3	<0.5	3	4	1	3	8
	Pakistani	<0.5	1	0	0	0	<0.5	0
	Bangladeshi	27	13	48	58	12	29	31
Betel nut/sopari chewed with no tobacco	Indian	4	2	4	1	2	5	7
	Pakistani	1	3	3	0	0	1	0
	Bangladeshi	35	28	39	36	24	47	43

Base: All Asian respondents

Passive smoking

Much of the contemporary debate about health risks associated with smoking centres around the effects of passive smoking. In particular, there has been extensive concern about the effects of smoking in the home on children. The UK-wide Health and Lifestyles Survey shows that almost all smokers smoke in their home, and that smoking in the home is in fact more widespread amongst smokers with children.

Amongst the African-Caribbean and South Asian communities, very high proportions also report to be smoking in the home (see Table 56). The only age group where smoking in the home is slightly reduced is amongst younger South Asians.

Table 56: Proportion of regular smokers, smoking at home (Source: AC Q183; AS Q138)

Demographic group	All adults				Standardised				UK population
	African-Caribbean %	Indian %	Pakis-tani %	Bangla-deshi %	African-Caribbean %	Indian %	Pakis-tani %	Bangla-deshi %	%
All	94	80	89	94	95	81	88	94	93
Women	89	*	*	*	92	*	*	*	95
16–29	87				91				90
30–49	92				90				96
50–74	100				100				98
Men	98	79	88	95	99	80	88	94	91
16–29	100	64	75	83	100	69	74	82	88
30–49	94	83	95	100	94	80	94	100	94
50–74	100	96	100	97	100	95	100	97	89

Base: All current regular smokers
*Bases for Asian women too small to be broken down

Table 56 shows that smoking in the home is widespread amongst African-Caribbean and South Asian households. Exposure to passive smoking was explored more widely in the next set of questions. All participants in the survey were asked if they spend any time in locations where they have to breathe in other people's cigarette smoke.

The UK-wide Health and Lifestyles Survey shows that over half of the UK population is regularly exposed to passive smoking. The African-Caribbean community reports very similar exposure rates, whilst those for South Asians are slightly lower (see Table 57). It is noticeable that African-Caribbean women report very high rates of exposure compared to the UK average, or to South Asian women. Whilst reported exposure rates decline across age groups amongst women of all ethnic groups, they remain very high amongst African-Caribbean women.

Amongst men, reported passive smoking exposure is highest amongst the UK sample. In general, reported exposure to passive smoking declines across age groups of men.

Table 57: Proportion of respondents who are exposed to others' cigarette smoke (Source: AC Q194; AS Q141)

Demographic group	All adults				Standardised				
	African-Caribbean %	Indian %	Pakis-tani %	Bangla-deshi %	African-Caribbean %	Indian %	Pakis-tani %	Bangla-deshi %	UK population %
All	59	44	43	50	58	44	44	48	55
Women	66	35	36	40	58	33	36	39	49
16–29	64	47	50	45	62	44	45	44	68
30–49	57	32	26	37	58	32	29	35	50
50–74	56	17	19	34	54	16	24	33	34
Men	58	53	51	59	57	55	53	58	66
16–29	59	70	61	74	61	70	64	73	75
30–49	66	52	49	58	65	52	52	59	64
50–74	47	32	35	36	50	37	35	37	42

Base: All respondents

Table 58 shows in more detail in which locations the different community groups are exposed to passive smoking. For the UK population the most frequently mentioned setting in which passive smoking is reported are pubs or restaurants (38%). This is followed closely by other social events (34%) and workplaces (31%).

For African-Caribbeans, other social events are most frequently mentioned (38%), followed by pubs and restaurants (29%), and work (25%).

Bangladeshis report the third-highest rate of exposure to passive smoking, after the UK population, and African-Caribbeans. For this group, the family home is the most frequently mentioned setting for passive smoking (29%). A further 27% mention other social events.

Pakistanis are most likely to mention other social events (24%), travelling (21%), and home (20%) as the main locations in which they are exposed to passive smoking. Finally, amongst Indians, other social events (22%), work (21%), and pubs or restaurants (20%), are mentioned as locations where sizeable sub-groups are exposed to passive smoking.

Table 58 also shows the variations in exposure to passive smoking in the various settings for each of the different demographic sub-groups. For most of the settings there is a consistent decline with age, and a higher rate of reported exposure amongst men than women. The exception here, as we have reported above, is African-Caribbean women, who report a slightly greater rate of exposure than African-Caribbean men.

Table 58: Proportion exposed to others' cigarette smoke in certain environments (Source: AC Q195; AS Q150)

		All	Women			Men		
			16–29	30–49	50–74	16–29	30–49	50–74
		%	%	%	%	%	%	%
Any place	UK population	55	68	50	34	75	64	42
	African-Caribbean	59	64	57	56	59	66	47
	Indian	44	47	32	17	70	52	32
	Pakistani	43	50	26	19	61	49	35
	Bangladeshi	50	45	37	34	74	58	36
In pubs/ restaurants	UK population	38	51	31	14	61	47	27
	African-Caribbean	29	28	20	10	37	45	29
	Indian	20	22	7	0	44	28	11
	Pakistani	10	11	0	0	16	14	11
	Bangladeshi	14	5	2	0	39	22	2
Other social events	UK population	34	48	27	17	54	39	25
	African-Caribbean	38	40	33	24	46	50	29
	Indian	22	24	11	4	44	27	18
	Pakistani	24	29	6	8	35	33	22
	Bangladeshi	27	16	12	0	52	41	22
At work	UK population	31	31	29	10	46	48	21
	African-Caribbean	25	20	32	21	32	30	13
	Indian	21	22	16	7	29	31	7
	Pakistani	16	15	1	0	27	32	9
	Bangladeshi	12	5	3	0	26	24	4
At home	UK population	23	35	23	15	32	23	16
	African-Caribbean	20	21	20	23	18	20	15
	Indian	12	21	15	5	12	7	6
	Pakistani	20	29	21	16	22	14	8
	Bangladeshi	29	39	34	34	29	15	22
While travelling	UK population	18	28	13	9	27	19	13
	African-Caribbean	17	24	16	17	14	27	8
	Indian	15	19	7	12	29	14	9
	Pakistani	21	31	8	7	30	25	14
	Bangladeshi	13	12	7	0	27	11	13
In shops	UK population	12	16	9	6	19	16	8
	African-Caribbean	15	14	16	10	17	17	13
	Indian	12	10	9	2	23	14	11
	Pakistani	15	15	5	4	20	25	16
	Bangladeshi	17	11	8	0	25	30	20

Base: All respondents

Table 59 shows the estimated amounts of time in an average day spent in inhaling other people's cigarette smoke. Very high exposure rates (five hours or more per day) are reported by 13% of the UK population. Those reported by all ethnic groups are lower.

The section at the bottom of Table 59 shows the average hours of exposure reported by those who inhale other people's smoke. Reported exposure is highest amongst the UK population (3.7 hours), followed by the Bangladeshi population (3.3 hours).

Table 59: Time spent inhaling others' cigarette smoke (Source: AC Q195; AS Q150)

			Women			Men		
		All %	16–29 %	30–49 %	50–74 %	16–29 %	30–49 %	50–74 %
None	UK population	45	32	50	66	24	36	58
	African-Caribbean	46	39	48	53	49	39	55
	Indian	58	55	70	83	32	51	69
	Pakistani	58	52	76	87	39	53	68
	Bangladeshi	52	58	65	68	27	44	68
Up to 1 hour	UK population	18	17	18	14	24	22	15
	African-Caribbean	21	30	26	24	14	12	12
	Indian	16	18	10	6	26	16	17
	Pakistani	14	16	14	10	17	13	10
	Bangladeshi	11	9	8	2	15	14	8
Over 1 hour –	UK population	10	13	8	5	12	13	8
up to 2 hours	African-Caribbean	7	5	3	4	9	10	9
	Indian	7	6	4	1	14	9	3
	Pakistani	8	11	2	0	9	8	17
	Bangladeshi	6	4	5	2	7	7	6
Over 2 hours –	UK population	12	16	12	7	18	14	9
up to 5 hours	African-Caribbean	13	13	14	9	13	18	13
	Indian	8	11	6	0	10	12	2
	Pakistani	8	9	3	0	17	11	2
	Bangladeshi	15	13	11	13	26	15	8
Over 5 hours	UK population	13	21	11	6	20	14	11
	African-Caribbean	9	8	8	9	12	11	9
	Indian	6	6	8	1	9	6	2
	Pakistani	7	9	2	3	9	9	1
	Bangladeshi	9	8	7	8	12	11	5
		(h)	(h)	(h)	(h)	(h)	(h)	(h)
Mean number	UK population	3.7	4.3	3.4	3.1	3.9	3.5	3.5
of hours	African-Caribbean	2.8	2.3	2.6	2.3	3.4	3.5	3.3
(Base: all	Indian	2.4	2.5	3.5	0.8	2.7	2.0	1.1
inhaling	Pakistani	2.6	2.9	2.0	2.1	2.7	3.1	1.6
others' smoke)	Bangladeshi	3.3	3.9	3.4	5.6	3.1	2.9	2.6

Base: All respondents

Perceived health effects

The vast majority of current regular smokers believe that their smoking has an effect on their health at the moment. Amongst the UK-wide sample, 13% feel that their smoking affects their health a great deal, and a further 32% say it influences their health a fair amount. Almost two in five (38%) report that their health is affected a little, and only 14% report that their health is not at all influenced.

Amongst the African-Caribbean and South Asian communities, a significantly higher proportion feel that their smoking currently affects their health a great deal. This is particularly so for Bangladeshis, where 27% feel their current health is affected a great deal by their smoking. African-Caribbean women also feel more strongly that their smoking affects their health at present. By contrast the proportion of African-Caribbean men who say their smoking does not affect their health at all is above the UK figure. This is also the case for Indian and Pakistani men.

Table 60: Perceived effects of smoking on health now (Source: AC Q190; AS Q145)

Affects health		All %	Women %	Men %
A great deal	UK population	13	12	14
	African-Caribbean	19	23	16
	Indian	18	*	19
	Pakistani	19	*	19
	Bangladeshi	27	*	26
A fair amount	UK population	32	33	30
	African-Caribbean	22	27	19
	Indian	19	*	18
	Pakistani	27	*	27
	Bangladeshi	24	*	25
A little	UK population	38	36	40
	African-Caribbean	26	28	25
	Indian	27	*	27
	Pakistani	27	*	28
	Bangladeshi	26	*	26
Not at all	UK population	14	16	12
	African-Caribbean	22	13	27
	Indian	22	*	22
	Pakistani	20	*	20
	Bangladeshi	15	*	16
Don't know	UK population	3	2	3
	African-Caribbean	11	9	12
	Indian	14	*	15
	Pakistani	6	*	5
	Bangladeshi	8	*	8

Base: All current regular smokers
*Bases too small for breakdown

All those who reported that their health is affected a great deal, a fair amount, or a little, were asked to describe what effect their smoking has on their health. In the UK-wide Health and Lifestyles Survey, the most frequently mentioned effect is breathlessness (43%), coughing (24%), and a general sense of being less fit (22%). There is some variation in the proportions mentioning the different respiratory problems amongst the African-Caribbean and South Asian communities. Bangladeshis are particularly likely to mention coughs (58%), and express a greater likelihood of getting chest infections (22%).

Table 61: Health effects of smoking (Source: AC Q191; AS Q146)

	All adults				Standardised				
	African-Caribbean %	Indian %	Pakis-tani %	Bangla-deshi %	African-Caribbean %	Indian %	Pakis-tani %	Bangla-deshi %	UK population %
Breathlessness	40	31	45	29	39	32	48	30	43
Coughing	33	40	38	58	34	41	36	57	24
Wheezing	9	5	4	6	9	4	4	6	7
Prone to chest infections	7	10	15	22	9	10	16	22	9
Less fit	18	25	26	13	15	26	27	12	22
Worry about serious illness	4	4	2	11	6	5	2	5	6

Base: All those who say smoking affects their health to some degree

Table 62 shows to what extent people feel their smoking is likely to affect their health in the future. Here a much more severe assessment of risk is provided; for the UK-wide survey 30% feel that their future health will be influenced a great deal. The proportions amongst the different black and South Asian communities who give the same answer are at least as great, if not greater. Again, Bangladeshis express the strongest concerns (41%).

Table 62: Perceived health effects of smoking in the future (Source: AC Q192; AS Q14)

Affects health		All %	Women %	Men %
A great deal	UK population	30	30	31
	African-Caribbean	35	45	28
	Indian	28	*	27
	Pakistani	37	*	37
	Bangladeshi	41	*	40
A fair amount	UK population	36	37	35
	African-Caribbean	32	28	34
	Indian	19	*	20
	Pakistani	27	*	26
	Bangladeshi	21	*	22
A little	UK population	17	17	17
	African-Caribbean	15	10	19
	Indian	13	*	13
	Pakistani	11	*	12
	Bangladeshi	10	*	11
Not at all	UK population	7	6	7
	African-Caribbean	4	5	4
	Indian	10	*	9
	Pakistani	11	*	11
	Bangladeshi	9	*	12
Don't know	UK population	10	10	9
	African-Caribbean	14	12	15
	Indian	30	*	31
	Pakistani	14	*	15
	Bangladeshi	18	*	18

Base: All current regular smokers
*Bases too small for breakdown

When asked, in the UK-wide Health and Lifestyles Survey, which health problems smokers feel they are most likely to encounter in the future, respiratory problems are again mentioned most frequently (e.g. chest infections or bronchitis was mentioned by 31%, problems with breathing or coughing by 30%). However, significant proportions also feel that their future health might be affected by lung cancer (26%), or heart disease (15%). It was one of the notable features of the UK-wide Health and Lifestyles Survey that such a high proportion of smokers feel that there is a considerable risk not only of their health being influenced in the future, but of encountering a major and possibly life-threatening disease.

A very similar pattern of response is found amongst the African-Caribbean and South Asian communities (see Table 63). Again respiratory or chest problems are mentioned by high proportions. References to lung cancer and heart disease also are high. Both African-Caribbean and Bangladeshi smokers mention lung cancer most frequently. Heart disease is significantly more likely to be mentioned by South Asian smokers.

Table 63: Future health effects of smoking (Source: AC Q193; AS Q148)

	All adults				Standardised				UK population
	African-Caribbean %	Indian %	Pakistani %	Bangladeshi %	African-Caribbean %	Indian %	Pakistani %	Bangladeshi %	%
Chest infections/bronchitis	25	35	23	29	23	36	23	30	31
Problems with breathing/coughing	26	23	16	14	23	25	20	13	30
Lung cancer	31	16	26	34	35	19	26	33	26
Breathlessness	18	21	19	12	13	23	22	12	20
Become less fit	12	12	15	20	9	12	15	18	16
Heart disease	17	20	26	27	19	24	32	26	15
Lung problems	12	5	10	11	13	7	13	11	9
Cancer (unspecified)	14	11	11	12	16	12	9	11	9
Other cancer	8	4	9	9	8	5	9	10	5
Get a serious illness	2	1	6	17	3	1	7	17	4
Other	8	8	14	10	10	9	14	9	3

Base: Those who think smoking will affect health in future

Smoking cessation

Table 64 shows the proportion in each of the communities, who have given up smoking (and who were previously regular cigarette smokers). Amongst the UK adult population, 22% are ex-regular smokers. More men, and particularly older men, have stopped smoking than women.

Amongst African-Caribbean, 10% of adults are ex-regular smokers, whilst amongst the South Asian communities much smaller proportions fall into this group.

It is possible to calculate a 'cessation rate' by dividing the proportion of ex-regular smokers by the sum of current and ex-regular smokers. In the UK-wide Health and Lifestyles Survey the cessation rate was 44%. Cessation rates are lower for the different black and minority communities (African-Caribbean 31%, Pakistani 29%, Indian 23% and Bangladeshis 15%). This clearly demonstrates that smoking cessation has been much less successful so far amongst the different black and minority ethnic communities, and that it is a particular problem amongst Bangladeshi smokers.

Table 64: Ex-regular cigarette smokers % (Source: AC Q167-169/177; AS Q122-124/132)

Demographic group	All adults				Standardised				UK population
	African-Caribbean %	Indian %	Pakis-tani %	Bangla-deshi %	African-Caribbean %	Indian %	Pakis-tani %	Bangla-deshi %	%
All	10	3	6	4	10	3	6	4	22
Women	8	0	<0.5	<0.5	8	0	<0.5	0	17
16–29	8	0	0	<0.5	8	0	0	0	8
30–49	7	0	1	0	7	0	1	0	17
50–74	8	0	0	0	9	0	0	0	24
Men	12	6	12	8	14	6	11	8	26
16–29	15	1	7	3	14	1	8	3	9
30–49	5	6	6	7	6	7	7	8	24
50–74	17	12	32	16	18	12	24	15	45

Base: All adults

The survey also provides evidence that smoking cessation is a much more recent phenomenon for smokers from African-Caribbean and South Asian communities. Table 65 shows that in the UK population, almost half gave up smoking longer ago than ten years. Around one in five gave up in the previous two years, 13% three to five years ago, and 23% six to ten years ago.

Amongst African-Caribbeans the proportion of ex-regular smokers who quit within the last two years rises to 33%; the same figure is found for Indian ex-regular smokers.

Both Pakistani and Bangladeshi ex-regular smokers report that they quit relatively recently; 45% of Pakistani ex-regular smokers, and 49% of Bangladeshi ex-regular smokers stopped smoking within the last two years. It must be remembered that these figures are based on a relatively small number of members of the different community groups. But whilst the total number of quitters is relatively small, the fact that so many of them are recent quitters may indicate some underlying shift towards smoking cessation.

Table 65: When gave up smoking (Source: AC Q173; AS Q128)

	All adults				Standardised				UK population
	African-Caribbean %	Indian %	Pakis-tani %	Bangla-deshi %	African-Caribbean %	Indian %	Pakis-tani %	Bangla-deshi %	%
In last 6 months	10	13	16	19	7	14	17	20	8
7–12 months ago	4	4	10	14	7	4	12	16	4
1–2 years	22	11	13	11	19	15	16	13	7
3–5 years	14	28	19	10	14	25	24	9	13
6–10 years	19	23	6	30	18	21	8	26	23
Longer ago	31	18	37	15	32	21	22	16	45

Base: Ex-regular smokers

Table 66 shows the number of attempts at cessation successful quitters made in order to give up smoking. In the UK-wide survey just over half of quitters managed to stop smoking on their first attempt. One in five took two attempts and a further 12% three to four attempts. Small proportions indicate a large number of unsuccessful attempts.

The figures for the black and minority ethnic communities are broadly in line, although there is an indication that fewer South Asians required very large numbers of attempts.

Table 66: Number of attempts to give up smoking before succeeding (Source: AC Q176; AS Q131)

	All adults				Standardised				UK population
	African-Caribbean %	Indian %	Pakis-tani %	Bangla-deshi %	African-Caribbean %	Indian %	Pakis-tani %	Bangla-deshi %	%
Mean number	4	2	3	2	3	3	2	2	3
Once	47	56	50	69	46	47	50	67	54
Twice	23	13	11	9	21	15	14	10	20
3–4 times	8	14	33	10	12	18	29	12	12
5–9 times	4	16	3	8	3	18	3	6	6
10–14 times	3	0	<0.5	0	2	0	1	0	4
15–19 times	0	0	0	0	0	0	0	0	<0.5
20+ times	12	0	3	0	6	0	1	0	3

Base: Ex-regular smokers

Successful quitters were also asked why they had given up smoking (Table 67). For all groups, including the national sample for the Health and Lifestyles Survey, health reasons are the main motivator. Amongst the UK-wide sample, general concerns about health or fitness are most frequently mentioned. Relatively few refer to specific advice from their doctor or, indeed, the diagnosis of a particular health problem.

Amongst South Asians the diagnosis of particular health problems, or direct advice from their GP, are much more frequently mentioned. This is particularly the case for Bangladeshis. It must be remembered that this group reports particularly high rates of respiratory and chest health problems and that, in addition, the reported housing conditions suggest high incidence of dampness, mould, and other housing factors which could aggravate respiratory problems.

For the UK population high proportions also mention the financial cost of smoking as a reason for giving up. Surprisingly, this does not appear to be such a major motivating factor for the black and minority ethnic communities.

Table 67: Reasons/motivations for giving up smoking (Source: AC Q174; AS Q129)

	All adults				UK population %
	African-Caribbean %	Indian %	Pakistani %	Bangladeshi %	
Health reasons					
Diagnosis of health problem	12	22	10	29	12
Advice from doctor	3	8	19	25	5
Pregnancy	10	0	0	0	7
General concern about health/fitness	26	30	32	20	37
More aware of health risks	21	13	6	14	15
Recommended by doctor	NA	0	14	8	NA
Financial					
Cost/save money	9	10	8	3	24
Cost of cigarettes went up	7	6	2	0	5
Social/work					
Pressure from family/friend	6	18	7	5	11
Religious reasons	4	3	6	3	NA
Can't smoke at work/no-smoking policy	0	3	2	0	1
Illness/death of relative/friend	4	0	3	0	7
Aesthetic/cosmetic`	2	0	0	3	3
Loss of enjoyment	6	3	2	0	NA
TV programme	1	0	0	3	5
New Year's resolution	4	0	4	0	1
Other	4	14	13	5	3
No specific reason	14	5	9	11	8

Base: Ex-regular smokers

Smoking cessation attempts amongst current regular smokers

The discussion of smoking cessation has so far focused on those who have succeeded in giving up smoking. It should be remembered that this is a very small proportion of the different black and minority ethnic communities, and that the gap between the proportion of quitters and smokers in these communities is much wider than the UK average.

Current regular smokers were asked a series of questions to assess their support and involvement in cessation activities. Table 68 confirms that the proportion of smokers who wish to quit smoking amongst the different black and minority ethnic communities is very similar to that of the UK population. Around two-thirds of smokers, irrespective of ethnic background, wish to give up smoking.

Table 68: Proportion of current regular smokers wishing to give up smoking (Source: AC Q184; AS Q139)

Demographic group	All adults				Standardised				
	African-Caribbean %	Indian %	Pakis-tani %	Bangla-deshi %	African-Caribbean %	Indian %	Pakis-tani %	Bangla-deshi %	UK population %
All	61	73	68	69	63	66	64	64	65
Women	65	*	*	*	65	*	*	*	65
16–29	70				70				73
30–49	54				56				67
50–74	80				67				54
Men	58	75	69	70	61	69	65	67	64
16–29	70	86	64	91	71	71	56	86	75
30–49	34	83	74	64	32	79	70	61	68
50–74	72	45	60	62	70	71	61	61	47

Base: All current regular smokers
*Bases too small for breakdown and standardisation for Asian women

An attempt was made to further assess to what extent those who wish to give up smoking have firm plans to quit. In the UK-wide Health and Lifestyles Survey the proportion of regular smokers who report to have firm plans to give up smoking is 29%. Table 69 would suggest that the desire to quit smoking may be slightly greater among black and minority ethnic communities.

Table 69: Proportion of current regular smokers who have firm plans to give up smoking (Source: AC Q185; AS Q140)

Demographic group	All adults				Standardised				UK population
	African-Caribbean %	Indian %	Pakis-tani %	Bangla-deshi %	African-Caribbean %	Indian %	Pakis-tani %	Bangla-deshi %	%
All	35	40	36	45	37	38	35	43	29
Women	32	*	*	*	36	*	*	*	32
16–29	33				38				39
30–49	26				25				31
50–74	57				57				27
Men	37	42	38	46	37	40	37	45	27
16–29	49	40	45	49	45	31	38	47	34
30–49	15	49	31	44	15	51	33	40	26
50–74	46	25	42	46	44	30	41	46	21

Base: All current regular smokers
*Bases for Asian women too small for further breakdown and standardisation

Other national research, such as the UK-wide Health and Lifestyles Survey, has shown that the vast majority of smokers have at some point tried to give up smoking. Given the very low rates of successful cessation reported earlier, one might assume that the proportion of smokers amongst black and minority ethnic communities who have tried to give up smoking would be very low. However, as Table 70 shows, around two-thirds of smokers in each of the different communities have at some point tried to give up smoking. Moreover, the number of attempts made to give up smoking is as high, and in some groups, slightly higher, than for the UK population at large.

Table 70: Proportion of current regular smokers who have tried to give up (Source: AC Q186; AS Q141)

Demographic group	All adults				Standardised				UK population
	African-Caribbean %	Indian %	Pakis-tani %	Bangla-deshi %	African-Caribbean %	Indian %	Pakis-tani %	Bangla-deshi %	%
All	62	68	69	67	65	70	69	65	81
Women	72	*	*	*	75	*	*	*	82
16–29	75				79				79
30–49	66				68				85
50–74	85				75				79
Men	54	69	69	68	57	73	70	67	81
16–29	40	57	75	75	41	66	74	76	81
30–49	54	80	68	53	53	80	66	54	84
50–74	68	70	64	74	66	72	69	73	76

Base: All current regular smokers
*Bases for Asian women too small for further breakdown and standardisation

Table 71 shows to what extent current smokers who have unsuccessfully tried to give up smoking, had any help or support in giving up smoking. The UK-wide survey shows that just over half of unsuccessful quitters had any help or support. Amongst the black and minority ethnic communities, African-Caribbeans who have not succeeded in quitting report the lowest use of any help or support, and Indians the highest.

Smokers who did not succeed in quitting in the UK-wide survey most frequently mention help and support from family, and smoking aids bought from the chemist as support used for trying to give up smoking.

Amongst the South Asian groups, social support is also frequently mentioned. This is particularly the case for Indian unsuccessful quitters.

Previous sections on cessation have suggested that medical advice appears to play a greater role amongst South Asian smokers. This is also born out by the figures in Table 71.

Other aids, such as nicotine replacement therapy or advice leaflets, are less frequently mentioned by the African-Caribbean, and Pakistani and Bangladeshi smokers who have unsuccessfully tried to give up smoking.

Table 71: Use of aids to give up smoking (Source: AC Q189; AS Q144)

	All adults				Standardised				
	African-Caribbean %	Indian %	Pakis-tani %	Bangla-deshi %	African-Caribbean %	Indian %	Pakis-tani %	Bangla-deshi %	UK population %
Help and support from family	13	30	19	17	15	32	21	17	22
Help and support from friends	10	11	16	10	8	13	18	11	15
Help and support at work	5	6	5	2	7	8	5	1	5
Advice from doctor	12	16	18	21	9	16	18	23	10
Prescription from doctor	1	11	7	1	2	10	8	2	5
Aid bought from chemist	7	16	11	6	7	17	10	6	21
Special clinic/group	<0.5	2	1	0	1	2	1	0	1
Advice booklets	6	13	6	1	4	14	7	1	14
Counselling	0	1	3	1	0	<0.5	3	1	1
Alternative treatments	0	0	1	0	1	<0.5	<0.5	1	5
None of these	64	41	49	53	65	37	48	52	46

Base: Current smokers who have tried to give up

The reasons given by unsuccessful quitters for starting to smoke again are broadly in line with those found in the UK-wide survey (Table 72). This survey shows that worries and stress, and a general lack of willpower are the most frequently cited factors for making people start smoking again. Lack of willpower is slightly more likely to be mentioned by Bangladeshis and Indians, whilst worries and stress are slightly more likely to be mentioned by African-Caribbeans and Pakistanis. There is also a sugges-tion that for Pakistanis and Indians, peer pressure is a significant factor for starting to smoke again.

Table 72: Factors which contributed to taking up smoking again (Source: AC Q188; AS Q143)

| | All adults | | | | Standardised | | | | |
	African-Caribbean %	Indian %	Pakis-tani %	Bangla-deshi %	African-Caribbean %	Indian %	Pakis-tani %	Bangla-deshi %	UK population %
Lack of willpower	27	42	35	46	26	41	35	48	32
Encouragement by friends/peer pressure	8	19	22	9	8	16	25	8	12
Worries/stress	34	22	35	13	32	21	21	13	35
Withdrawal symptoms	5	7	9	17	5	8	11	17	10
Loss of enjoyment	6	9	11	12	7	10	12	11	7
Weight gain	1	4	4	3	1	4	4	3	5
Loss of social props	8	3	4	3	6	4	5	3	7
Nothing in particular	5	5	9	6	5	3	6	5	5

Base: Current smokers who have tried to give up

Workplace smoking policy

Workplaces have been targeted as a major setting for health promotion activities. The UK-wide Health and Lifestyles Survey shows that as far as employees are concerned, limited progress has been made in the provision of either designated smoking areas or complete no-smoking areas, or in helping smokers to quit smoking.

For example, only half of the working population covered in the Health and Lifestyles Survey report the presence of no-smoking signs in their workplace (Table 73), and only 30% mention leaflets and posters about how to stop smoking being made available at their place of work.

Provision is even more limited for more interactive interventions. Only 7% of employ-ees mention that advice from doctors or personnel is available, 4% mention that their workplace provides advice from outside counsellors or self-help groups, and 3% report that their place of work runs stop smoking groups.

The survey of African-Caribbeans shows slightly higher proportions mentioning no-smoking signs or leaflets and posters, and similar proportions mentioning other provision for smokers. South Asians employees are much less likely to report the availability of information materials, or any interactive advice or counselling.

Table 73: Smoking provision at work (Source: AC Q199; AS Q152)

	All adults				Standardised				
	African-Caribbean %	Indian %	Pakis-tani %	Bangla-deshi %	African-Caribbean %	Indian %	Pakis-tani %	Bangla-deshi %	UK population %
Leaflets/posters on how to stop smoking	40	17	19	24	37	15	20	22	30
No-smoking signs	61	39	34	34	56	35	29	32	51
A smoking room	29	15	21	12	27	13	17	11	28
Advice from doctors/personnel	11	3	5	3	9	3	5	2	7
Advice from outside counsellors/contact with self-help groups	2	3	1	2	3	3	1	1	4
Work with trade unions to promote smoking bans	7	4	3	2	5	3	3	2	6
Run stop smoking groups	2	3	2	3	1	2	2	4	3
Support from management to reduce work stress	3	3	1	0	3	2	1	0	1
Time-off for counselling or treatment	2	2	1	0	2	1	1	0	2

Base: All working but not self-employed

The UK-wide survey shows that 18% of employees work in workplaces where smoking is banned completely, and that 54% work in workplaces where smoking is allowed in special sections only; 28% work in workplaces where smoking is allowed anywhere.

The figures for African-Caribbean workers show that slightly higher proportions work in workplaces with a complete smoking ban, or where smokers and non-smokers are segregated. For this group, only 18% work in workplaces where smoking is allowed everywhere. Table 74a shows the degree to which smoking is allowed in particular workplace locations, such as catering areas (24% of African-Caribbeans say it is allowed to smoke in this area), or customer or visitor areas (12%).

Table 74a: Smoking restrictions in the workplace (African-Caribbeans) (Source: AC Q197–Q199)

Smoking	African-Caribbean %	UK population %
Completely banned	22	18
Allowed everywhere	18	28
Allowed in special sections only	60	54
Allowed in open work areas	6	6
Allowed in private offices	11	18
Allowed in catering/eating areas	24	19
Allowed in conference/meeting areas	10	15
Allowed in customer/visitor areas	12	15

Base: All African-Caribbeans working but not self-employed

The use of a differently worded questionnaire for the Asian samples makes a full comparison between South Asian workers, African-Caribbean and workers surveyed in the UK-wide survey difficult. The only comparative item concerns workplaces with a complete ban on smoking. As Table 74a shows, in the UK-wide survey, 18% of workers report a complete ban on smoking in their workplace, and 22% of African-Caribbeans report the same at their place of work. Amongst South Asians, broadly similar proportions of Indians (15%) and Pakistanis (19%) report a complete smoking ban (Table 74b). Bangladeshis, however, are much less likely to report a complete ban on smoking (6%).

Table 74b: Smoking restrictions in the workplace (Asians) (Source: AS Q152)

	Indian	Pakistani	Bangladeshi
Complete ban on smoking	15	19	6
Smoking allowed in private offices only	13	11	13
Smoking allowed in catering/eating area only	14	15	13
Smoking allowed in customer/visitor area only	3	2	5

Base: Asians working but not self-employed

6. Health promotion

Health promotion activities

The survey included a detailed section about health education or health promotion provided through the primary health care setting. Table 75 shows which health promotion topics GPs or other members of the primary health care team have discussed with women from the different black and minority ethnic communities. The table also shows the data obtained from the UK-wide Health and Lifestyles Survey.

In the UK-wide survey child health is mentioned most frequently (19%), followed by contraceptive advice (18%), weight loss (16%), and healthy food (12%).

For African-Caribbean women, weight loss is mentioned as the most frequent topic of discussion with the primary health care team (22%), followed by child health (15%), contraception (13%) and stress (13%). Overall, similar proportions of African-Caribbean women (65%) report to have discussed any health promotion topics in the past 12 months (the comparative UK figure is 68%).

South Asian women are less likely to report to have had health promotion discussions with members of the primary health care team in the past 12 months. Amongst Indian and Bangladeshi women, 46% report to have had some form of health education advice or discussion, and amongst Pakistani women the figure is 40%.

For Indian women, the most frequently mentioned topics are healthy food and weight loss (15% each), for Pakistani women weight loss (15%) and child health (12%), and for Bangladeshi women child health (19%) and healthy food (10%). It is noticeable that Indian women are less likely than any other group of women to mention child health.

South Asian women are less likely to mention having had discussions about contraception at their GP surgery. The higher reported incidence of the use of family planning clinics combined with the reduced rate of discussion with GPs would therefore suggest that a number of South Asian women prefer to discuss family planning issues at a clinic rather than their surgery.

Table 75: Topics discussed by women with member of staff in last year (Source: AS Q70; AC Q103)

	All women				UK population
	African-Caribbean %	Indian %	Pakistani %	Bangladeshi %	Women %
Children's health	15	10	12	19	19
Contraception	13	7	6	8	18
Losing weight	22	15	15	6	16
Healthy food	11	15	9	10	12
Stress	13	7	8	6	11
Childhood immunisation	10	5	4	8	9
Smoking	4	1	0	1	6
Exercise/fitness	4	5	3	2	5
Emotional problems	2	1	2	2	3
Heart disease	3	4	3	3	3
Cancer	2	0	0	2	3
Alcohol	1	1	0	0	1
HIV/AIDS	0	0	0	0	<0.5
None of these	35	54	60	54	32

Base: Those who have been to surgery in last 12 months

Table 76 shows the health education topics discussed by men with members of the primary health care team. The UK-wide survey showed that men are significantly less likely than women to discuss health education issues at surgery. The overall figures for men from the different ethnic minority communities are broadly similar to those found in the UK-wide survey.

In the UK-wide survey the key topics mentioned by men are healthy food (13%), weight loss (12%) and physical activity (11%).

The topics mentioned for African-Caribbean men are broadly similar to those identified in the UK-wide survey.

Amongst Pakistani and Bangladeshi men, physical activity is mentioned much less frequently. Bangladeshi men are particularly likely to have discussed smoking, children's health, and heart disease with their GP or other members of the primary health care team.

Table 76: Topics discussed by men with member of staff in last year (Source: AS Q70; AC Q103)

	All men				UK population
	African-Caribbean %	Indian %	Pakistani %	Bangladeshi %	Men %
Healthy food	9	12	12	15	13
Losing weight	15	16	9	6	12
Exercise/fitness	8	8	6	3	11
Smoking	7	3	7	12	9
Stress	8	6	7	5	9
Heart disease	3	7	5	10	8
Children's health	1	8	7	11	6
Alcohol	4	4	0	0	4
Childhood immunisation	1	1	2	3	2
Contraception	1	2	1	2	2
Cancer	0	0	0	1	2
Emotional problems	2	1	1	1	1
HIV/AIDS	1	0	1	1	1
None of these	57	58	63	54	56

Base: Those who have been to surgery in last 12 months

Members of the South Asian communities were asked which health promotion topics they found easy to discuss with their GP and which ones they found difficult. Table 77 shows the proportions who described discussion with their GP either as easy or difficult. In addition there are proportions who were undecided, or could not answer the questions since the issue had not arisen in their experience. The issues are ordered by the ratio of people who describe discussion with their GP as easy over those who describe it as difficult.

The topic which generally is seen as the easiest one to discuss with general practitioners is children's health. Both men and women feel that this is an unproblematic area.

Similarly, weight control is generally seen as an uncontentious issue.

Discussions about smoking and alcohol also receive a positive ratio. Amongst women, discussions of alcohol or smoking are of relatively low salience (as expressed by the low numbers who give an opinion); amongst men the salience is somewhat greater, especially for smoking. Indian men are also more likely to express an opinion on discussions about alcohol consumption.

An issue which appears of relevance to South Asians is stress. Here, again, the majority of South Asians describe discussions about stress or worries as unproblematic. But the proportion who describe such discussions as difficult increases, with about one in seven women, and one in nine men describing such discussions as difficult.

Similarly, discussion of mental and psychological problems is seen as somewhat more difficult, with Bangladeshis particularly likely to describe such discussions with their GP as difficult.

The area in which communication with a GP appears to be most problematic is over issues concerning sexual health. High proportions of South Asians express a difficulty in discussing with their GP contraception, gynaecological problems, sexual problems, or HIV/AIDS. Again, it is Bangladeshis who are most likely to express such problems.

Table 77: Ease of discussing issues (Source: AS Q113)

		Women			Men		
		Indian %	Pakis-tani %	Bangla-deshi %	Indian %	Pakis-tani %	Bangla-deshi %
Children's	Easy	64	73	73	60	51	66
health	Difficult	2	4	4	2	3	2
Weight control	Easy	70	82	68	74	83	78
	Difficult	7	7	11	5	5	7
Alcohol	Easy	23	21	8	43	30	19
	Difficult	3	5	8	4	3	3
Smoking	Easy	23	25	12	39	46	44
	Difficult	3	4	8	3	4	8
Stress	Easy	46	57	50	58	64	58
	Difficult	12	14	17	8	12	13
Mental/	Easy	43	58	38	49	63	45
psychological	Difficult	17	19	22	16	15	18
Contraception	Easy	45	50	42	43	48	44
	Difficult	14	21	28	9	15	15
HIV/AIDS	Easy	28	33	18	41	41	28
	Difficult	11	17	20	9	13	14
Gynaecological	Easy	67	65	45	NA	NA	NA
	Difficult	21	26	40	NA	NA	NA
Emotional	Easy	30	50	29	40	51	36
problems	Difficult	24	25	31	21	22	21
Sexual	Easy	28	39	15	41	43	34
problems	Difficult	21	28	40	16	20	27

Base: All respondents

Tables 78a–g provide further insights into GP-based health promotion activities. They show the proportions of each community who discussed a particular health promotion issue with different members of staff in the primary health care team, the extent to which they found this discussion useful, and the follow-up activities provided. It should be noted that these tables are based on very small bases and that comparisons should therefore be undertaken with some caution.

A number of broad findings emerged from these tables. Firstly, across all community groups, the key providers of health promotion activities are GPs. In the UK-wide sample, smaller proportions also mentioned an involvement by the practice nurse. This is also the case for the African-Caribbean sample, but amongst South Asians, the role of the practice nurse is much more restricted to the point where, amongst Bangladeshis, health promotion advice is more or less the exclusive domain of general practitioners.

Those who report to have received health promotion advice generally describe it as useful (for example in the UK-wide survey, evaluations vary from 52% who describe discussions on smoking as useful to 87% who describe discussions about contraception as useful).

It is difficult to identify any specific patterns as far as the follow-up activity to health promotion discussions is concerned. This is further complicated by the relatively small numbers who report to have received any specific health promotion advice. Broadly speaking, there would appear to be a reliance on the use of printed materials such as leaflets, booklets, or diet sheets. Use of such materials is more limited amongst South Asians, especially Bangladeshis where availability of mother-tongue materials as well as literacy limit the choice of available materials. The data would also suggest that general practitioners are less likely to recommend physical activity to South Asians.

Table 78a: Health promotion discussed: diet (Source: AS Q71-73; AC Q104-106)

	All adults				UK population %
	African-Caribbean %	Indian %	Pakistani %	Bangladeshi %	
Discussed					
– GP	7	12	9	12	8
– Nurse	3	1	2	<0.5	4
– Health visitor	<0.5	<0.5	<0.5	<0.5	<0.5
– Midwife	0	0	<0.5	<0.5	<0.5
– Dietitian	1	1	1	<0.5	1
– Other	0	<0.5	<0.5	0	<0.5
Base: All been to surgery					
Discussion thought to be useful	86	78	89	89	81
Follow-up activity					
– keep a diary	14	5	13	9	7
– given leaflets/booklets	25	20	25	20	33
– advice on diet	34	22	17	31	NA
– diet sheet to lose weight	20	7	7	5	40
– referred to specialist	3	3	11	2	5
– take more exercise	26	19	13	12	30
– fitness plan	7	5	1	5	6

Base: All who discussed healthy food

Table 78b: Health promotion discussed: weight loss
(Source: AS Q74–76; AC Q107–109)

	All adults				UK population %
	African-Caribbean %	Indian %	Pakistani %	Bangladeshi %	
Discussed					
– GP	16	12	11	6	10
– Nurse	4	2	1	<0.5	4
– Health visitor	<0.5	<0.5	<0.5	0	<0.5
– Midwife	0	<0.5	<0.5	0	<0.5
– Dietitian	1	1	<0.5	<0.5	<0.5
– Other	<0.5	1	<0.5	0	<0.5
Base: All been to surgery					
Discussion thought to be useful	75	73	63	82	76
Follow-up activity					
– special diary	8	7	6	4	6
– leaflets/booklets	20	18	20	12	20
– advice on diet	8	21	21	33	NA
– diet sheet	29	17	16	15	34
– take more exercise	20	22	30	37	30
– fitness plan	1	5	9	1	5
– referred to specialist	5	1	10	0	6
– clinic recommended	9	7	1	1	3

Base: All who discussed weight loss

Table 78c: Health promotion discussed: heart disease
(Source: AS Q89-91; AC Q122-124)

	All adults				UK population %
	African-Caribbean %	Indian %	Pakistani %	Bangladeshi %	
Discussed					
– GP	2	5	4	6	5
– Nurse	0	<0.5	<0.5	0	1
– Health visitor	0	0	0	0	0
– Midwife	0	0	0	0	0
– Dietitian	0	0	0	0	0
– Other		<0.5	0	0	0
Base: All been to surgery					
Discussion thought to be useful	71	86	79	84	84
Follow-up activity					
– leaflets/booklets	6	25	11	5	12
– diet sheet	14	15	21	10	12
– referred to specialist	4	23	44	23	19
– take more exercise	0	23	10	8	25
– reduce weight	9	9	17	3	27
– reduce smoking	8	4	9	22	20
– special diary	0	0	7	0	3
– clinic recommended	8	7	9	0	4

Base: All who discussed heart disease

Table 78d: Health promotion discussed: exercise/fitness
(Source: AS Q77-79; AC Q110-112)

	All adults				UK population %
	African-Caribbean %	Indian %	Pakistani %	Bangladeshi %	
Discussed					
– GP	5	5	4	2	6
– Nurse	<0.5	1	1	<0.5	2
– Health visitor	0	0	0	0	<0.5
– Midwife	0	0	0	0	<0.5
– Physiotherapist	<0.5	0	1	0	<0.5
– Other	0	<0.5	0	0	<0.5
Base: All been to surgery					
Discussion thought to be useful	83	75	57	74	75
Follow-up activity					
– special diary	6	0	20	9	3
– referred to specialist	5	4	13	13	8
– clinic recommended	5	0	0	11	2
– fitness plan	29	5	18	26	18
– take more exercise	22	14	22	11	29
– leaflets/booklets	8	15	9	0	15
– diet sheet	18	9	16	0	15
– recommend joining health/sports club	0	2	16	0	4

Base: All who discussed exercise/fitness

**Table 78e: Health promotion discussed: stress/worries
(Source: AS Q86–88; AC Q119–121)**

	All adults				UK population %
	African-Caribbean %	Indian %	Pakistani %	Bangladeshi %	
Discussed					
– GP	10	6	7	5	9
– Nurse	<0.5	<0.5	1	0	<0.5
– Health visitor	0	<0.5	<0.5	<0.5	<0.5
– Midwife	0	0	0	0	<0.5
– Counsellor	<0.5	0	0	0	<0.5
– Other	0	0	<0.5	0	<0.5

Base: All been to surgery

Discussion thought to be useful	68	67	74	68	75
Follow-up activity					
– special diary	3	1	9	5	4
– leaflets/booklets	14	8	13	19	7
– take exercise	12	6	5	14	15
– recommend to join class/support group	9	0	0	7	6
– referred to specialist	11	10	25	0	12
– clinic recommended	5	6	5	0	5

Base: All who discussed stress/worries

Table 78f: Health promotion discussed: smoking (Source: AS Q83–85; AC Q116–118)

	All adults				UK population %
	African-Caribbean %	Indian %	Pakistani %	Bangladeshi %	
Discussed					
– GP	4	1	4	6	6
– Nurse	<0.5	<0.5	<0.5	0	1
– Health visitor	0	0	0	0	<0.5
– Midwife	0	0	0	0	<0.5
– Dietitian	0	0	0	0	0
– Other	<0.5	0	0	0	0
Base: All been to surgery					
Discussion thought to be useful	78	45	72	84	52
Follow-up activity					
– special diary	0	11	8	5	4
– leaflets/booklets	22	20	10	13	21
– clinic recommended	5	6	2	3	3
– nicotine substitutes recommended	17	3	17	7	20
– referred to specialist	10	2	4	0	3
– class/support group recommended	6	6	2	0	4

Base: All who discussed smoking

Table 78g: Health promotion discussed: contraception
(Source: AS Q92–94; AC Q125–127)

	All adults				UK population %
	African-Caribbean %	Indian %	Pakistani %	Bangladeshi %	
Discussed					
− GP	5	4	3	4	9
− Nurse	<0.5	<0.5	<0.5	1	1
− Health visitor	0	<0.5	<0.5	0	<0.5
− Midwife	<0.5	0	0	0	<0.5
− Dietitian	0	0	0	0	0
− Other	0	0	<0.5	0	<0.5

Base: All been to surgery

Discussion thought to be useful	94	94	95	89	87
Follow-up activity					
− special diary	21	5	0	3	2
− leaflets/booklets	43	22	22	11	16
− free condoms	9	5	26	10	4
− referred to specialist	1	7	3	9	7
− referred to clinic	14	12	37	41	7

Base: All who discussed contraception

Use of other health information sources

The previous sections have shown that primary health care teams only have a limited impact in the provision of health information advice. Table 79 shows to what extent members of the different ethnic minority communities use other information sources. The first set of data in Table 79 shows the proportions of the different communities who report to have used a range of different information sources. In the second set of data in the table these information sources are aggregated into generic groupings. The last set of findings from the table, at the bottom, shows the proportions of each community who report not to have used any of the listed information sources.

It is worthy of comment that significant minorities of the South Asian community have not come across any health information in any of the sources (most of which are mass media sources) listed. Amongst Indians, one in four report not to have encountered any health information in any of the listed sources. This increases slightly to around three in ten Pakistanis, and increases even further to over two in five Bangladeshis.

Looking at the individual sources, television is most frequently mentioned. It features most strongly amongst African-Caribbeans (69%) but falls back in importance amongst South Asians, particularly Bangladeshis, where fewer than 30% mention health information advice on television.

The second most important item are leaflets obtained at GP surgeries. Again, African-Caribbeans are most likely to mention this as an information source. Use declines across the different South Asian groups, with Bangladeshis, again, reporting the lowest usage.

Sizeable minorities mention information obtained from magazines. Again, African-Caribbeans are more likely to mention such sources, followed by Indians and Pakistanis, with Bangladeshis reporting the lowest incidence.

Interactive advice from GPs or from community advisers is mentioned less frequently. However, here the gap between the different ethnic minority communities is much less pronounced, and Bangladeshis report a similar incidence to that reported by other South Asian groups.

Organisations involved in the provision of health promotion advice have been keen to champion the use of community radio stations and of videotapes. So far, only small minorities of the different black and minority ethnic communities report having used such sources for health information advice. These sources are most frequently mentioned by African-Caribbeans, followed by Indians. Bangladeshis, again, report the lowest exposure rates.

The generic aggregation in the second half of the table shows that written materials are the key information source for each of the four ethnic communities. Television and video are of some importance, particularly amongst African-Caribbeans, but have less impact amongst South Asians at the moment. Across all the different community groups, there is very little awareness of health information advice provided via radio broadcasts.

Table 79: Use of health information sources (Source: AS Q114; AC Q156a)

	Women				Men			
	African-Caribbean %	Indian %	Pakis-tani %	Bangla-deshi %	African-Caribbean %	Indian %	Pakis-tani %	Bangla-deshi %
Television programme	69	41	34	25	69	47	39	30
Leaflets from GP	67	40	38	28	54	41	31	27
Information in magazines	49	22	20	12	31	24	23	14
Advice from GP/ community worker	25	18	11	18	25	18	17	17
Information in national newspapers	26	13	8	7	29	18	18	12
Information in local/community newspapers	19	16	9	7	18	15	15	11
National radio	14	10	10	3	22	13	13	4
Local/community radio	14	12	8	4	14	16	8	5
Leaflets in shops	21	10	7	1	12	8	9	6
Video for use at home	4	5	3	3	6	3	4	1
Any written information	87	56	47	35	79	60	55	43
Leaflets	74	45	40	29	58	43	35	32
TV/video	70	42	36	26	70	48	40	30
Radio	23	20	16	7	28	24	18	8
None	0	26	33	44	0	22	25	42

Base: All adults

Future issues for health promotion

The current survey has identified a considerable gap in the provision of information about health for the different black and minority ethnic communities. Consistently, the Bangladeshi community shows poor access to the various information sources.

The final part of this report tries to assess to what extent health information advice is of relevance to the different South Asian communities (this question was not included on the questionnaire for African-Caribbeans), and what linguistic strategies should be used by information providers.

Table 80 shows that across the different South Asian communities and also across gender, there is a considerable interest in health education advice. Overall, two-thirds of South Asians express an interest in at least one of the different health education issues listed in Table 80.

The most frequently mentioned topic is a healthy diet, mentioned by around a third of South Asian women and a similar proportion of South Asian men. This is followed by physical activity, mentioned by one in five women, and one in four men. Children's health is a further topic of interest to significant proportions of women, and slightly lower proportions of men.

Another important topic of interest to South Asians is strategies for coping with stress or pressure.

For men, heart disease also is of interest, and amongst Pakistani and Bangladeshi men smoking cessation.

Many of the other critical health education themes appear to be of much less salience to South Asians. Relatively few mention an interest in contraception, sex education, STDs, or HIV/AIDS. Similarly, there is only limited interest in further information about alcohol consumption or drugs.

Table 80: Health education topics of interest (Source: AS Q112; AC Q155)

	Women			Men		
	Indian %	Pakistani %	Bangladeshi %	Indian %	Pakistani %	Bangladeshi %
Healthy eating	37	30	36	37	29	32
Physical exercise	21	21	19	24	25	24
Children's health	23	19	27	15	12	16
Coping with stress/pressure	19	16	19	18	15	18
Heart disease	8	8	9	18	13	13
Stopping smoking	1	2	4	8	13	16
Advice on contraception/ birth control	5	4	6	4	3	3
Menstruation/periods	6	5	6	3	0	0
HIV/AIDS	3	3	2	4	4	4
Drugs	1	4	0	3	3	4
Sexually transmitted diseases	2	3	0	3	2	4
Drinking alcohol	1	1	0	7	1	0
Sex education	1	3	0	1	1	1
Nothing	33	41	36	36	35	40

Base: All respondents

Chapter 2 covers in considerable detail the linguistic and literacy skills of the different communities. A clear limitation for the provision of any written materials is the proportion of people who are completely illiterate. Table 81 shows the language preference for the provision of written material, based on those who can read. It is apparent that any information targeted at the different communities needs to be bilingual. Whilst the majority of young people prefer to have advice provided in English, middle-aged and older sections of the community generally prefer mother-tongue materials. This is particularly the case for Pakistanis and Bangladeshis.

The critical languages in which materials therefore should be provided are English, Urdu, Bengali, Gujerati, and Punjabi.

Table 81: Language prefer to read about health advice (Source: AS Q116)

Ethnic group		All %	Women 16–29 %	Women 30–49 %	Women 50–74 %	Men 16–29 %	Men 30–49 %	Men 50–74 %
Indian	English	62	80	51	16	90	67	37
	Gujerati	26	16	33	41	5	28	37
	Punjabi (Sikh or Gurmukhi script)	16	7	21	33	6	14	26
	Hindi	7	5	6	20	3	10	5
Pakistani	English	60	77	22	0	86	59	41
	Urdu	48	31	73	71	20	63	62
	Punjabi (Urdu or Perso-Arabic script)	4	2	7	6	1	4	10
Bangladeshi	English	47	58	11	6	85	42	16
	Bengali	68	59	90	100	32	79	96

Base: All adults

Table 82 identifies in which languages members of the different South Asian communities prefer to receive health information advice on television or radio. As with the provision of written materials, the preference for English is primarily found amongst younger people. Mother-tongue provision becomes more important amongst the middle-aged and older members of the communities, and in addition, preferences for regional dialects such as Sylheti are being expressed.

Table 82: Language prefer to listen to health advice on television or radio (Source: AS Q115)

Ethnic group		All %	Women 16–29 %	Women 30–49 %	Women 50–74 %	Men 16–29 %	Men 30–49 %	Men 50–74 %
Indian	English	63	83	50	26	90	67	46
	Gujerati	27	17	35	45	11	28	27
	Punjabi	19	9	23	29	8	21	29
	Hindi	15	10	13	31	5	21	31
Pakistani	English	50	68	15	1	85	53	39
	Urdu	54	42	71	69	29	67	61
	Punjabi	22	16	33	54	9	18	30
Bangladeshi	English	39	51	5	4	78	39	22
	Bengali	60	56	71	65	32	70	80
	Sylheti	23	18	40	52	10	18	24

Base: All adults

References

Badger, F., Atkin, K., Griffiths, R. (1982) 'Why don't general practitioners refer their disabled patients to district nurses?' *Health Trends*, **21**, 31–2.

Balarajan, R. and Bulusu, L. (1990) 'Mortality among immigrants in England and Wales, 1979–1983', in OPCS, 1990.

Balarajan, R. and Raleigh, V. S. (1993) *Ethnicity and Health: a Guide for the NHS*. Department of Health.

Balarajan, R. and Yuen, P. (1986) 'British smoking and drinking habits: variations by country of birth', *Community Medicine*, **8**, 237–9.

Balarajan, R., Yuen, P. and Raleigh, V. S. (1989) 'Ethnic differences in general practitioner consultation', *British Medical Journal*, **59**, 668–70.

Ball, S. S. (1987) 'Psychological symptomatology and health beliefs in Asian patients', in Dent, H. (ed.) *Clinical Psychology: Research and Development*. Croom Helm.

Bhopal, R. S. (1986) 'The inter-relationship of folk, traditional and Western medicine within an Asian community in Britain', *Social Science and Medicine*, **22**, 99–105.

Blakemore, K. (1983) 'Ethnicity, self-reported illness and use of medical services by the elderly', *Postgraduate Medical Journal*, **59**, 668–70.

Blaxter, M. (1985) 'Self-definition of health status and consulting rates in primary care', *Quarterly Journal of Social Affairs*, **1**, 131–71.

Blaxter, M. (1990) *Health and Lifestyles*. Tavistock/Routledge.

Brown, C. (1984) *Black and White Britain: the Third PSI Survey*. Heineman-Educational.

CHELFHSA/MORI 1993 *East London Health*. CHELFHSA London.

Cruickshank, J. K. (1993) 'The challenge for the Afro-Caribbean community in controlling stroke and hypertension', in *The Health of the Nation – The Ethnic Dimension*. North East Thames/North West Thames RHA/Department of Health.

Cruickshank, J. K., Cooper, J., Burnett, M., MacDuff, J. and Drubra, U. (1991) 'Ethnic differences in fasting plasma C-peptide and insulin in relation to glucose tolerance and blood pressure', *Lancet*, **338**, 842–7.

Department of Health (1992a) *On the State of the Public Health: the Annual Report of the Chief Medical Officer of the Department of Health for the Year 1991*. HMSO.

Department of Health (1992b) *The Health of the Nation: a Strategy for Health in England.* HMSO.

Donaldson, L. J. and Clayton, D. H. (1984) 'Occurrence of cancer in Asians and non-Asians', *Journal of Epidemiology and Community Health*, **38**, 203–7.

East London & City Health Authority/MORI (1994) *Evaluation of Bilingual Health Advocacy Services.* East London & City Health Authority, London.

Ebrahim, S., Patel, N., Coasts, M., Creig, C., Grilley, J., Banham, C. and Stacey, S. (1991) 'Prevalence and severity of morbidity among Gujerati elders: a controlled comparison, *Family Practice*, **8**, 57–62.

Gillam, S. J., Jarman, B., White, P. and Law, R. (1989) 'Ethnic differences in consultation rates in urban general practice', *British Medical Journal*, **299**, 953–7.

Health Education Authority (1994a) *Health-related Resources for Black and Minority Ethnic Groups.* Health Education Authority.

Health Education Authority (1994b) 1992 Health and Lifestyles Surveys. HEA.

Hyndman, S. J. (1990) 'Housing, dampness and health amongst British Bengalis in East London', *Social Science and Medicine*, **30**(1), 131–41.

Jain, C., Narayan, N. and Narayan, P. (1985) 'Attitudes of Asian patients in Birmingham to general practitioner services', *Journal of the Royal College of General Practitioners*, **35**, 416–18.

Johnson, M. R. D. (1986) 'Inner city residents, ethnic minorities and primary health care in the West Midlands', in Rathwell, T. and Phillips, D. (eds) *Health, Race and Ethnicity.* Croom Helm.

Jones, T. (1993) *Britian's Ethnic Minorities: an Analysis of the Labour Force Survey.* PSI.

Knight, T. M., Smith, Z., Lockton, J. A., Sahota, P., Bedford, A., Toop, M., Kernohan, E. and Baker, M. R. (1993) 'Ethnic differences in risk markers for heart disease in Bradford and implications for preventative strategies', *Journal of Epidemiology and Community Health*, **47**, 89–95.

McAvoy, B. R. and Raza, R. (1988) 'Asian women: (i) contraceptive knowledge, attitudes and usage, (ii) contraceptive services and cervical cytology', *Health Trends*, **20**, 11–17.

McCormick, A., Rosenbaum, M. and Fleming, D. (1990) 'Socio-economic characteristics of people who consult their general practitioner', *Population Trends*, **59**, 8–10.

McKeigue, P. M., Ferrie, J. E., Pierpoint, T. and Marmot, M. G. (1993) 'Association of early-onset coronary heart disease in South Asian men with glucose intolerance and hyperinsulinemia', *Circulation*, **87**, 152–61.

McKeigue, P. M. and Marmot, M. G. (1991) 'Obesity and coronary risk factors among South Asians', *Lancet*, **337**, 972.

McKeigue, P. M., Marmot, M. G., Adelstein, A. M., Hunt, S. P., Shipley, M. J., Butler, S. M., Riemersma, R. A. and Turner, P. R. (1985), 'Diet and risk factors for coronary heart disease in Asians in North-West London, *Lancet*, **ii**, 1086–90.

McKeigue, P. M., Marmot, M. G., Syndercombe Court, Y. D., Cottier, D. E., Rahman, S. and Riemersma, R. A. (1988) 'Diabetes, hyperinsulinaemia and coronary risk factors in Bangladeshis in East London', *British Heart Journal*, **60**, 390–6.

National Consumer Council (1993) *Consumer Concerns 1993: Consumers' Views on Aspects of Health Services*. NCC Publications.

National Co-ordinating Network (1994) *First Five Years of the NHS Cervical Screening Programme*. Anglia and Oxford Regional Health Authority.

Norman, A. (1985) *Triple Jeopardie: Growing Old in a Second Homeland*. Centre for Policy on Ageing.

Nzegwu, F. (1993) *Black People and Health Care in Contemporary Britain*. International Institute for Black Research, Reading.

OPCS (1990) *Mortality and Geography: the Registrar General's Decennial Supplement for England and Wales*. HMSO.

Stubbs, M. (1985) *The Other Languages of England: Linguistic Minorities Project*. Routledge & Kegan Paul, 1985.

Wright, C. (1983) 'Language and communication problems in an Asian community', *Journal of the Royal College of General Practitioners*, **33**, 101–4.

Appendix. Example questionnaire

English language version of questionnaire
for Asian respondents

BEM Health & Lifestyle Survey 1992
Asian Questionnaire 21/9/92

Sample point number ☐☐☐☐☐☐ WRITE IN NUMBERS FROM TOP OF CONTACT SHEET
(20)(21)(22)(23)(24)(25)

(19–25)
SKIP 26

INTERVIEWER: START HERE WITH INTRODUCTION AND DEMOGRAPHICS
MORI is carrying out this survey for the Health Education Authority and it is a major study on the nation's health. But before I ask any questions about health issues, I need to check some more details about yourself and your household, to make sure we interview people from all backgrounds. All the information you give me is confidential.

Gender (27)
Female.......................1
Male.......................2   27

Age (28)
16–24 1
25–34 2   **Exact Age**
35–44 3   WRITE IN
45–54 4
55–64 5   ☐☐
65+ 6   (29) (30)

Q1 How many people are there usually living here — that includes yourself, any other adults and children?

1 2 3 4 5 6 7 8 9 10 11 12+   31

Q2 Are there any children aged 15 or under in this household?
Yes...........1 ASK Q3
No ....2 GO TO Q4   32

ASK IF YES
Q3 CODE NUMBERS OF CHILDREN IN EACH AGE GROUP
0–1   1 2 3 4+   33
2–3   1 2 3 4+   34
4–5   1 2 3 4+   35
6–10   1 2 3 4+   36
11–12   1 2 3 4+   37
13–15   1 2 3 4+   38

ASK ALL
Q4 Does this household own this accommodation or do you rent it?
(39)
Owned outright 1
Owned/being bought on mortgage ..2
Rented from council 3
Rented from housing association ...4
Rented from private landlord 5
Other (WRITE IN & CODE '6')........
..................................6   39

Q5 Phone in Household (40)
Yes 7
No 8
Tel No._____   40

Q6a How many rooms does this accommodation have? Please include all rooms

☐ ☐
(41) (42)   41/42

Q6b And how many bedrooms does this accommodation have?

☐
(43)   43

Q6c Do you have a kitchen used by your household only?
(44)
Yes 1
No....................2   44

Q6d Do you have a toilet used by your household only?
(45)
Yes 1
No....................2   45

Q6e Do you have a bathroom used by your household only?
(46)
Yes 1
No....................2   46

I/we confirm that I/we have conducted this interview face–to–face with the person named on the contact sheet for the address number given above and that I/we asked all the relevant questions and recorded the answers in conformance with the survey specifications and within the MRS Code of Conduct.

Date of interview   _____

Interviewer Number: ☐☐☐☐/☐ Interviewer Signature:_____
(47)(48)(49)(50) (51)

Interviewer Number: ☐☐☐☐/☐ Interviewer Signature:_____
(52)(53)(54)(55) (56)

(47–56)

Q7   SHOWCARD A   What forms of heating do you use regularly in cold weather? MULTICODE OK

Central heating: (57)

Mains gas 1
Bottled gas 2
Fuel oil 3
Electricity   – normal tariff 4
                  – off peak 5
Solid fuel   – smokeless 6
                  – non–smokeless 7

Non–central heating:

Mains gas fire/convector 8
Fan heaters 9
Electric bar fires 0
Storage heaters X
Calor/Butane gas heaters . . . . Y
                                               (58)
Paraffin heaters 1
Oil filled electric
   radiator 2
Solid fuel open grate 3
Solid fuel stove/
   enclosed grate 4
Other (WRITE IN & CODE 5) . . . .

. . . . 5   57/
Don't know 6   58

Q8   INTERVIEWER   OBSERVATION
        (CODE BY OBSERVATION)

     Address is:

     House/bungalow
                                               (59)
     –   detached 1
     –   semi–detached/
            end of terrace 2
     –   mid–terrace 3

     Maisonette 4
     Flat 5
     Rooms/bedsitter 6
     Other (WRITE IN & CODE '7') . . .

     7   59

Q9   FRONT DOOR IS ON:
                                               (60)
     Ground floor/street–level 1
     Low–rise (1st or 2nd floor) 2
     Mid–rise (3 to 6th floor) 3
     High–rise (7 floors or higher) . . 4   60

Q10   Do you own a car or have use of a car?
                                               (61)
     Own car 1
     Use of car (eg company car) . . 2
     No car 3   61

Q11   And do you personally have a full driver's licence, or not?
                                               (62)
     Yes 1
     No 2

Q12   How would you describe your race or ethnic origin? DO NOT PROMPT. CODE BELOW
                                               (63)
     Black British 1
     Afro–Caribbean 2
     West Indian 3
     Guyanese 4
     Black African 5
     Nigerian 6
     Ghanaian 7
     Zambian 8
     Indian 9
     Pakistani 0
     Bangladeshi X
     Bengali . . . . Y
                                               (64)
     Punjabi 1
     East African Asian 2
     Other (WRITE IN & CODE 3) . . . . .

     3

     No opinion 4   63/
     Refused 5   64

     ASK ALL
Q13a In what country were you born?
                                               (65)
     West Indies/Guyana 1
     India 2   GO TO
     Pakistan 3
     Bangladesh 4
     Kenya 5
     Uganda 6   Q14
     Tanzania 7
     Zambia 8
     Malawi 9
     Nigeria 0
     Ghana X
     Other Africa (WRITE IN &
        CODE 'Y') . . . .

     . . . . Y
                                               (66)
     Northern Ireland 1   ASK
     England, Wales 2   Q13b
     Scotland 3
     Other country (WRITE IN &
        CODE '4')
                                               65/
     4   66

IF BORN IN BRITAIN ASK Q13b
Q13b And in what country were your parents born? MULTICODE OK

(67)

West Indies/Guyana	1
Indian	2
Pakistan	3 GO
Bangladesh	4
Kenya	5 TO
Uganda	6
Tanzania	7
Zambia	8 Q14
Malawi	9
Nigeria	0
Ghana	X
Other Africa (WRITE IN & CODE 'Y')	
	Y

(68)

Northern Ireland	1 ASK
England, Wales	2 Q13c
Scotland	3 GO TO
Other country (WRITE IN & CODE '4')	Q14
	4

67/
68

IF BOTH PARENTS BORN IN BRITAIN ASK Q13c
Q13c And in what country were your Grandparents born? MULTICODE OK

(69)

West Indies/Guyana	1
Indian	2
Pakistan	3
Bangladesh	4
Kenya	5
Uganda	6
Tanzania	7
Zambia	8
Malawi	9
Nigeria	0
Ghana	X
Other Africa (WRITE IN & CODE 'Y')	
	Y

(70)

Northern Ireland	1
England, Wales	2
Scotland	3
Other country (WRITE IN & CODE '4')	
	4

69/
70

ASK ALL
Q14 Which languages do you speak including English? CODE ALL MENTIONS

ASK IF MORE THAN ONE MENTIONED AT Q14. (IF ONE LANGUAGE ONLY, SEE Q18)
Q15 Which do you consider is your main spoken language? SINGLE CODE ONLY

Q16 Which do you speak at home? MULTICODE OK

Q17 Which do you speak at work? MULTICODE OK

	Q14 Speak (71)	Q15 Main (72)	Q16 At home (73)	Q17 At work (74)
English	1	1	1	1
Bengali	2	2	2	2
Gujerati	3	3	3	3
Hindi	4	4	4	4
Kutchi	5	5	5	5
Panjabi	6	6	6	6
Sylheti	7	7	7	7
Urdu	8	8	8	8

Other (WRITE IN & CODE 9)

(Q14) 9

....

(Q15) 9

....

(Q16) 9

....

(Q17) 9

71/
74

....

Don't work 0

ASK IF ENGLISH NOT CODED AT Q14. OTHERS GO TO Q20

Q18 How well would you say you understand English when it is spoken to you?
READ OUT

Q19 How well would you say you speak English? READ OUT

	Q18 Understand (75)	Q19 Speak (76)
Very well	1	1
Fairly well	2	2
A little	3	3
Not at all	4	4

75/
76

ASK ALL

Q20 Which languages do you read? CODE ALL MENTIONS

ASK IF MORE THAN ONE MENTIONED AT Q20. (IF ONE LANGUAGE ONLY SEE Q22)

Q21 Which language do you consider is the main language you prefer to read?
SINGLE CODE ONLY

	Q20 Read (77)	Q21 Main (78)
English	1	1
Bengali	2	2
Gujerati	3	3
Hindi	4	4
Panjabi (Urdu or Perso–Arabic Script)	5	5
Panjabi (Sikh or Gurmukhi Script)	6	6
Urdu	7	7
Other (WRITE IN & CODE 8)		
(Q20)	8	
....		
(Q21)		8
....		
None of these	9	9 GO TO Q24

77/
78

IF ONLY ONE LANGUAGE CODED AT Q20 AND IT IS <u>NOT</u> ENGLISH, ASK Q22.
ASK ABOUT MAIN LANGUAGE READ AT Q21 (CODES 2–8) BUT NOT ENGLISH

Q22 How well would you say you read ....(LANGUAGE)? READ OUT

	(79)
Very well	1
Fairly well	2
A little	3

79

ASK ALL WHO READ ENGLISH (CODE 1 AT Q20)

Q23 How well would you say you read English? READ OUT

	(80)
Very well	1
Fairly well	2
A little	3

CARD 2   10

ASK ALL

Q24   What is your religion or church?

	(11)
Baptist	1
Buddhist	2
Islam/Muslim	3
Sikhism	4
Hinduism	5
Church of England/Wales/ Scotland/Ireland	6
Roman Catholic	7
Methodist	8
Seventh Day Adventist	9
Jehovah's Witness	0
Pentecostal/Church of God/ Church of Christ	X
Cherubim and Seraphim	Y
Rastafarian	1
	(12)
Jewish	2
Other (WRITE IN & CODE '3')	
....	3
None	4
Don't know	5

11/
12

Q25   Which of these best describe you? READ OUT

		(13)
1.	Married	1
2.	Single	2
3.	Living with partner	3
4.	Divorced/separated but living with a partner	4
5.	Divorced/separated and not living with a partner	5
6.	Widowed	6

13

ASK ALL EXCEPT THOSE IN SINGLE PERSON HOUSEHOLDS (CODE 1 AT Q1) WHO GO TO Q28

Q26   I would now like to ask a few questions about you and your household and the jobs that you do. First of all, including yourself, how many adults aged 16+ are there in this household? USE LEADING ZERO

☐ ☐
(14) (15)

14/
15

Q27 **What relationship is each one to you?**

IF MORE THAN 8, USE CONTINUATION SHEET

	Respondent (Person 1) (16)	16+ YEARS ONLY PERSON NUMBER						
		2 (17)	3 (19)	4 (21)	5 (23)	6 (25)	7 (27)	8 (29)
Respondent	1							
Spouse/partner		2	2	2	2	2	2	2
Daughter/son		3	3	3	3	3	3	3
Daughter in-law/son-in-law		4	4	4	4	4	4	4
Father/mother		5	5	5	5	5	5	5
Father-in-law/mother-in-law		6	6	6	6	6	6	6
Grandparent/in-law		7	7	7	7	7	7	7
Grandchild/in-law		8	8	8	8	8	8	8
Brother/sister/in-law		9	9	9	9	9	9	9
Aunt/uncle/in-law		0	0	0	0	0	0	0
Cousin/in-law		X	X	X	X	X	X	X
Nephew/niece/in-law		Y	Y	Y	Y	Y	Y	Y
		(18)	(20)	(22)	(24)	(26)	(28)	(30)

Other (WRITE IN & CODE 1)

16/30

.... 1 1 1 1 1 1 1

ASK FOR EACH ADULT AGED 16+ IN HOUSEHOLD, STARTING WITH RESPONDENT (IF MORE THAN 8, USE CONTINUATION SHEET)

Q28 SHOWCARD B **Which statement on this card applies to each person aged 16+ in the household, starting with you?**

(IF SINGLE ADULT HOUSEHOLD, SAY: **Which statement on this card applies to you?**)

	Respondent (Person 1) (31)	PERSON NUMBER						
		2 (33)	3 (35)	4 (37)	5 (39)	6 (41)	7 (43)	8 (45)
Paid employee working full-time(30+ hrs/week)	1	1	1	1	1	1	1	1
Paid employee working part-time(up to 29 hrs/week)	2	2	2	2	2	2	2	2
Self-employed working full-time	3	3	3	3	3	3	3	3
Self-employed working part-time	4	4	4	4	4	4	4	4
Retired with occupational pension or other private income	5	5	5	5	5	5	5	5
Retired on state benefits only	6	6	6	6	6	6	6	6
Unemployed for less than 6 months	7	7	7	7	7	7	7	7
Unemployed for more than 6 months	8	8	8	8	8	8	8	8
At school	9	9	9	9	9	9	9	9
Other full-time education	0	0	0	0	0	0	0	0
On government training scheme	X	X	X	X	X	X	X	X
Temporarily sick/disabled less than 6 months	Y	Y	Y	Y	Y	Y	Y	Y
	(32)	(34)	(36)	(38)	(40)	(42)	(44)	(46)
Long term sickness/disabled (6 months or longer)	1	1	1	1	1	1	1	1
Looking after home or family	2	2	2	2	2	2	2	2
Other	3	3	3	3	3	3	3	3

31/46

ASK ABOUT CURRENT JOB FOR EACH PERSON WORKING (CODES 1–4 AT Q28)
FOR EACH PERSON RETIRED (CODES 5–6 AT Q28), ASK ABOUT PREVIOUS JOB
FOR EACH PERSON UNEMPLOYED LESS THAN 6 MONTHS (CODE 7 AT Q28), ASK
ABOUT PREVIOUS JOB
IF NOBODY IN HOUSEHOLD CODED 1–7 AT Q28, GO TO Q31

Q29   What is/was the name or title of your/his/her job?

PROBE FOR TITLE/GRADE.

ASK IF RESPONSIBLE FOR MANAGING ANY STAFF; IF YES, HOW MANY.

IF SELF–EMPLOYED, ASK IF ANY STAFF EMPLOYED; IF YES, HOW MANY.

Respondent (Person 1)	47/49
Person 2	50/52
Person 3	53/55
Person 4	56/58
Person 5	59/61
Person 6	62/64
Person 7	65/67
Person 8	68/69

Q30   What kind of work do/did you (etc) do most of the time? PROBE: Do/did you (etc) use any machinery or special skills? IF YES: What? | Card 3 | 10

CHECK SPECIAL SKILLS/TRAINING

Respondent (Person 1)	11/13
Person 2	14/16
Person 3	17/19
Person 4	20/22
Person 5	23/25
Person 6	26/28
Person 7	29/31
Person 8	32/34

ASK ALL

Q31a SHOWCARD C   **Please look at this card and tell me which, if any, is the highest educational qualification you have obtained in this country?**

		(35)
01	CSE/GCE 'O' level/GCSE/Scottish 'O' Grade/ Scottish Standard Grade	1
02	GCE 'A' level/Scottish Higher Grade/ Scottish Certificate of Sixth Year Studies (CSYS)....................	2
03	Recognised trade apprenticeship completed	3
04	Clerical and commercial qualifications (eg typing/ shorthand/book-keeping/commerce).........................	4
05	City and Guilds Certificate – Operative	5
06	City and Guilds Certificate – Craft/Intermediate/ Ordinary/Part 1....................................	6
07	City and Guilds Certificate – Advanced/Final/Part II	7
08	City and Guilds – Full Technological (FTC)/ Part III................................	8
09	Insignia Award in Technology (GCIA)	9
10	JIB/NHC or other Craft Technician Certificate.....................	0
11	ONC/OND (or SNC/SND) or TEC/BEC/BTEC (or SCOTEC/ SCOBEC/SCOTVEC) National/General Certificate or Diploma	X
12	HNC/HND (or SHNC/SHND) or TEC/BEC/BTEC (or SCOTEC/SCOBEC/SCOTVEC) Higher or Higher Cert or Diploma	Y

		(36)
13	Nursing qualifications (eg SEN, SRN, SCM) – including Nursery Nursing (NNEB)	1
14	Polytechnic (or Central Institute) Diploma or Certificate (NOT CNAA VALIDATED)	2
15	University or CNAA Diploma or Certificate – including Dip HE and Teaching Training College Certificate	3
16	University or CNAA First Degree – including B Ed	4
17	University or CNAA Post Graduate Diploma	5
18	University or CNAA Higher Degree – MSc, PhD, etc.................	6
19	Professional qualification – membership awarded by professional institution	7
20	Any other qualifications (WRITE IN & CODE '8')	
	....	8
99	No formal qualifications	9
	Don't know	0

35/
36

Q31b **And have you received any educational qualifications outside of Britain? IF YES: What is the highest you have received?**

....

....

....

37/
38

HEALTH CONCERNS

Q32 Now I would like to ask you some questions about your health, thinking first about your health in general. How do you feel about your health? Would you say that for your age your health is . . .

READ OUT. ALTERNATE ORDER. TICK START

(39)

Very good 1	
Fairly good 2	
Fairly poor 3	
Very poor 4	
Don't know 5	**39**

Q33 Are you suffering from any illness?

(40)

Yes . . . . 1 ASK Q34a AND b

No . . . . 2 GO TO Q34c　　　**40**

Q34 (a) What is the matter with you? PROBE IN DETAIL What else? IF UNCLEAR ASK: What do you mean by that? WRITE IN

. . . .

. . . .

. . . .

. . . .

. . . .　　**41/**

. . . .　　**42**

(b) Has this stopped you doing things?

(43)

Yes 1

No . . . . 2　　**43**

ASK ALL
(c) Do you do anything in particular to keep or improve your health?

(44)

Yes . . . . 1 ASK Q34d

No . . . . 2 GO TO Q35　　**44**

ASK IF YES
(d) What are the most important things you do?
PROBE FOR 3. WRITE IN ON SEPARATE LINES

1 – . . . .　　**45/47**

2 – . . . .　　**48/50**

3 – . . . .　　**51/53**

ASK ALL

Q35 SHOWCARD D   Here is a list of health issues which can affect people's health. **Which, if any, of these are having a bad effect on your health <u>at the moment</u>? Just read out the numbers of those you worry about. MULTICODE OK**

Q35
Current risk
(54)

1.	The kind of food I eat	1
2.	The quality of my housing	2
3.	The amount I smoke	3
4.	Worries at home	4
5.	Living on my own	5
6.	The amount of alcohol I drink	6
7.	My weight	7
8.	The amount of exercise that I do	8
9.	Pollution where I live	9
10.	Pollution where I work	0
11.	Pollution in general	X
12.	Worries at work	Y

(55)

13.	My sexual behaviour	1
14.	Road traffic in this area	2
15.	Being unemployed	3
16.	The amount of violent crime in this area	4
17.	The amount of racism in this area	5
	Other (WRITE IN & CODE 6)	
	....	6
	None of these	7
	Don't know	8

54/
55

Q36 SHOWCARD E   And which, if any, of these illnesses and health problems have you **personally ever suffered from? Just call out the numbers. MULTICODE OK**

Q36
(56)

1.	Severe arthritis/rheumatism	1
2.	Breathing difficulties eg bronchitis	2
3.	Cancer	3
4.	Depression/anxiety/nerves	4
5.	Alcoholism	5
6.	Stroke	6
7.	HIV/AIDS	7
8.	Heart disease	8
9.	Back pain	9
10.	STDs (sexually transmitted diseases)	0

(57)

11.	Anorexia nervosa	X
12.	Sickle Cell	Y
13.	High blood pressure	1
14.	Stomach problems eg ulcer	2
15.	Diabetes	3
16.	Thalassaemia	4
	Other (WRITE IN & CODE 5)	
	....	5
	None of these	6
	Don't know	7

56/
57

ENVIRONMENT

ASK ALL

Q37a **I would like to ask you a few questions about your neighbourhood. Would you say this neighbourhood ... READ OUT. ROTATE ORDER. TICK START**

(58)

☐   **Is a place where you personally feel safe** 1
     or not? 2
     Neither/don't know 3

     has things for young children
       – playgrounds and parks for example 4
     or not? 5
     Neither/don't know 6

     has good local transport 7
     or not? 8
     Neither/don't know 9

☐   **has good leisure things for people like**
       yourself – leisure centres or community
       centres for example 0
     or not? X
     Neither/don't know .... Y   58

Q37b **SHOWCARD F Which of these problems affect you in your neighbourhood?   Just call out the numbers of the ones you think apply.**

(59)

1   The amount of road traffic......................... 1
2   Car exhaust fumes 2
3   Industrial fumes and emissions 3
4   Litter and rubbish 4
5   The level of crime and vandalism 5
6   The level of noise................................ 6
7   The amount of racial abuse or violence 7

     Other (WRITE IN & CODE 8) ....

     8

     None of these 9
     Don't know 0   59

Q37c **SHOWCARD G Thinking about your own home now, which if any of the items on this card do you think are a risk to your physical health or mental well–being? Just call out the numbers of the ones you think.**

(60)

1   Lack of heating 1
2   Dampness... 2
3   Condensation..................................... 3
4   Mould 4
5   The general maintenance of your home 5
6   Not enough space in your home 6
7   The quality of the drinking water 7
8   Lack of soundproofing or level of noise 8

     Other (WRITE IN & CODE 9) ....

     9

     None of these 0
     Don't know X   60

CHECK IF RESPONDENT IS WORKING (F/T OR P/T) AT Q28

WORKING 1   ASK Q37d
NOT WORKING 2   GO TO Q38

Q37d IF WORKING, ASK
SHOWCARD H Thinking now about the work you do, which if any of the things on this list do you think are a risk to your own physical health or mental well—being? Just call out the numbers of the ones you think apply.

(61)

1	The materials you have to handle	1
2	The equipment you have to use	2
3	Industrial fumes and emissions	3
4	The level of noise................................	4
5	Worries at work	5
6	The number of hours you work.....................	6
7	Racial abuse at work	7
8	Sexual harassment at work........................	8

Other (WRITE IN AND CODE 9) ....

....9

None of these....................................0
Don't know X

61

PSYCHO–SOCIAL HEALTH

<u>ASK ALL</u>
Q38 SHOWCARD I **This card lists a number of things which may have happened to you. Could you tell me please which, if any, of these have happened to you in the past 12 months? You can just call out the number.**

ASK FOR EACH ONE MENTIONED
Q39 SHOWCARD J **And could you tell me please, from this card, how worrying you found . . . (EVENT). REPEAT FOR EACH EVENT MENTIONED**

	Q38	Q39 Degree of Worry					
	Events (62)	Very worrying	Fairly worrying	Not very worrying	Not at all worrying	Don't know	
1 – Serious illness or injury 1		1 .... 2 .... 3 ....4 5					64
2 – Serious illness or injury of someone close to you 2		1 .... 2 .... 3 ....4 5					65
3 – Death of a close relative or friend 3		1 .... 2 .... 3 ....4 5					66
4 – Problems at work 4		1 .... 2 .... 3 ....4 5					67
5 – Losing your job/retirement 5		1 .... 2 .... 3 ....4 5					68
6 – Another member of this household losing their job 6		1 .... 2 .... 3 ....4 5					69
7 – Changing your job 7		1 .... 2 .... 3 ....4 5					70
8 – Personal experience of theft, mugging, break–in or another crime 8		1 .... 2 .... 3 ....4 5					71
9 – Verbal abuse due to your race or colour 9		1 .... 2 .... 3 ....4 5					72
10 – Physical attack due to your race or colour 0		1 .... 2 .... 3 ....4 5					73
11 – Discrimination at work or anywhere else due to your race or colour X		1 .... 2 .... 3 ....4 5					74
12 – Divorce, separation or break–up of an intimate relationship .... Y (63)		1 .... 2 .... 3 ....4 5					75
13 – Problems with your existing partner 1		1 .... 2 .... 3 ....4 5					76
14 – Pregnancy 2		1 .... 2 .... 3 ....4 5					77
15 – Problems with children 3		1 .... 2 .... 3 ....4 5					78
						CARD 4	10
16 – Problems with parents or close relatives 4		1 .... 2 .... 3 ....4 5					11
17 – Moving home.................5		1 .... 2 .... 3 ....4 5					12
18 – Financial difficulties 6		1 .... 2 .... 3 ....4 5					13
19 – Problems with neighbours 7		1 .... 2 .... 3 ....4 5					14

None of these 8   GO TO
Don't know 9   Q40

ASK ALL
Q40 SHOWCARD K   **Which, if any, of the things on this card do you usually do to cope with worry? Just call out the numbers of the ones which apply. PROBE: Which others?**

		(15)
1	Try not to think about it	1
2	Discuss it with a close friend	2
3	Discuss it with a relative	3
4	Work harder to occupy myself	4
5	Take more exercise/more physical activity	5
6	Go to pub/have a drink	6
7	Smoke more	7
8	Drink more	8
9	Eat more	9
10	Pray/meditate	0
11	Get help and advice from a doctor	X
12	Get prescription from doctor	Y

(16)

13	Get help and advice from counsellor or advice organisation	1
14	Spend more time thinking about my problems	2
15	Spend more time going out with friends or relatives	3
16	Never have any worry	4
	None of these	5
	Don't know	6

15/
16

SOCIAL SUPPORT

ASK ALL
Q41   How long have you lived In this area (within ten minutes walk of your home)?

                                                   (17)

Less than 12 months	1
1 year	2
2 years	3
3 years	4
4 years	5
5–9 years	6
10–14 years	7
15–19 years	8
20 years or more	9
Don't know	0

17

Q42   Apart from the people you live with, do you have any other relatives whom you speak to or see regularly?

  (18)

Yes	1
No	2

18

Q43   And do you have any friends whom you speak to or see regularly?

(19)

Yes	1
No	2

19

Q44   SHOWCARD L   From this card, could you tell me please which, If any, of these you have done In the past fortnight? MULTICODE OK

(20)

1	Went to visit relatives	1
2	Had relatives visit me	2
3	Went out with relatives	3
4	Spoke to relatives on the phone	4
5	Went to visit friends	5
6	Had friends visit me	6
7	Went out with friends	7
8	Spoke to friends on the 'phone	8
9	Spoke to neighbours	9
10	Spoke to a health professional (eg doctor, nurse, midwife, health visitor)	0
11	Attended an adult education or night school class	X
12	Participated in a voluntary group or local community group	Y

(21)

13	Participated In community or religious activities	1
14	Went to a leisure centre	2
15	Went to another social outing (PLEASE SPECIFY & CODE 3)	
	....	3
	None of these	4

20/
21

Q45 SHOWCARD M **If you needed help and advice, which, if any, of the people on this card could you discuss personal issues with. Please give me the numbers that apply**

		(22)
1	Partner or spouse	1
2	Female relatives	2
3	Male relatives	3
4	Female friends	4
5	Male friends	5
6	Girlfriend	6
7	Boyfriend	7
8	Neighbours	8
9	Community worker	9
10	Community leader	0
11	Social worker	X
12	Counsellor/therapist	Y
13	Priest or clergy or religious leader	1
14	Home help	2
		(23)
15	Meals–on–wheels	3
16	Family doctor/GP	4
17	Nurse	5
18	Midwife	6
19	Health visitor	7
	Someone else	
	(PLEASE SPECIFY & CODE 8)	
	. . . .	8
	None of these	9

22/
23

HEALTH SERVICES

Q46 **Are you currently registered with a doctor or GP?**

	(24)
Yes................................1	ASK Q47
No 2	
Don't know........................3	GO TO Q60 (p18)

24

IF REGISTERED WITH DOCTOR/GP ASK Q47

Q47 **Are you registered with this doctor on the National Health Service or privately?**

| | (25) |
| NHS................................1 |
| Private............................2 |
| Both...............................3 |
| Don't know........................4 |

25

Q48 **Is the doctor or GP you normally see male or female?**

| | (26) |
| Male...............................1 |
| Female ....2 |
| It varies..........................3 |
| Don't know........................4 |

26

Q49 **Which would you prefer to see if you had the choice, a male or female doctor or GP?**

| | (27) |
| Male...............................1 |
| Female ....2 |
| No preference ....3 |
| Don't know........................4 |

27

Q50 SHOWCARD N   **Which of these best describes your doctor?**

| | (28) |
| White..............................1 |
| Asian..............................2 |
| Chinese............................3 |
| African ....4 |
| West Indian ....5 |
| Other (WRITE IN & CODE 6)........... |
| ....6 |
| It varies..........................7 |
| Don't know........................8 |

28

DO NOT ASK Q51–Q57 IF ENGLISH IS MAIN OR ONLY LANGUAGE AT Q20–21 (GO TO Q58).

Q51   In what language do you and your doctor normally speak to each other?

(29)

English 1
Bengali 2
Gujerati 3
Hindi 4
Kutchi 5
Panjabi 6
Sylheti 7
Urdu 8
Other (WRITE IN AND CODE 9)

. 9

Have Interpreter with me/provided 0
Don't know X   29

Q52   How easy or difficult is it for you and your GP/doctor to understand each other?
READ OUT

(30)

Very easy 1
Fairly easy 2
Fairly difficult 3
Very difficult 4
No opinion 5   30

Q53   When you see your doctor, do you ever have someone there to interpret, or not?

(31)

Yes . . . . 1 ASK Q54
No . . . . 2 GO TO Q57   31

ASK IF YES

Q54   Do you ever take someone with you to act as an interpreter?

(32)

Yes . . . . 1 ASK Q55
No . . . . 2 GO TO Q56   32

ASK IF YES

Q55   Would that person be your . . . ? READ OUT

(33)

Husband/wife 1
Mother/father (in—law) 2
Son/daughter (in—law) 3
Another family member 4
A friend 5
Other (WRITE IN & CODE 6)

. 6
It varies 7   33

Q56 ASK ALL WHO USE AN INTERPRETER AT Q53. OTHERS GO TO Q58.
Does your doctor/GP ever provide someone who can act as an interpreter?

          (34)
Yes 1   GO TO Q58
No 2   ASK Q57   34

Q57 ASK ALL WHO DON'T USE INTERPRETER AT Q56
Is that because you don't need an interpreter, or because no–one is available to interpret, or for some other reason?

          (35)
Interpreter not needed 1
No interpreter available 2
Other (WRITE IN & CODE 3) . . . .

. 3

Don't know 4   35

Q58 ASK ALL
How easy or difficult is it for you to get to your doctor's/GP's surgery?
READ OUT ALTERNATE ORDER. TICK START

          (36)
Very easy 1   GO TO Q60
Fairly easy 2
Fairly difficult 3   ASK Q59
Very difficult 4
Don't know 5   GO TO Q60   36

Q59 ASK IF DIFFICULT (CODES 3–4 AT Q58)
Why do you find it difficult to visit your doctor's/GP's surgery? MULTICODE OK

          (37)
Surgery hours are inconvenient 1
Too far away 2
Poor public transport 3
Difficult to park the car 4
Situated in high crime area 5
Poor access for disabled/elderly etc. . . .6
Difficulty in walking 7
Other (WRITE IN & CODE 8) . . . .

. 8

Don't know 9   37

Q60 ASK ALL
When did you last visit a doctor's/GP's surgery or health centre for your own health? I am interested in any visit you may have made for yourself, not necessarily to see a GP.

          (38)
In last week 1
Over 1 week, within last month 2
Over 1 month, within last 2 months 3   ASK
Over 2 months, within last 4 months . . .4   Q61
Over 4 months, within last 6 months . . .5
Over 6 months, within last 12 months . .6
Over 1 year, within last 3 years 7
Over 3 years, within last 5 years 8   GO
Over 5 years, within last 10 years 9
Over 10 years 0   TO
Can't remember .X
Never . . . . .Y   Q111 (p38)   38

Q61 ASK IF CODES 1–6 AT Q60 (OTHERS GO TO Q111)
How many times have you visited a surgery for your own health over the last 12 months? Again I'm interested in any visit you may have made for yourself, not necessarily to see a GP.

WRITE IN ☐☐

(39) (40)

39/
40

I would now like to ask you some questions about the last occasion that you visited the surgery or health centre for your own health, (<u>not</u> the last time you accompanied someone else)

Q62 SHOWCARD O   When you last visited the surgery or health centre, which of these people did you see and talk to? Who else? MULTICODE OK

	(41)
Doctor/GP	1
Practice Nurse	2
Physiotherapist	3
Health visitor	4
Midwife	5
Practice pharmacist	6
Receptionist	7
Social worker	8
Counsellor	9
Dietician	0
Other (WRITE IN AND CODE X)	
..................................X	
None of these	Y

41

Q63 Did you make an appointment in advance to see any one of the staff or health professionals there, or did you just turn up, or were you asked to attend?

	(42)
Made an appointment	1
Just turned up	2
Asked to attend	3
Other (WRITE IN & CODE 4)	
....	4
Can't remember	5

42

Q64　　SHOWCARD P　**Why did you go to the surgery or health centre?**　MULTICODE OK

(43)

1	To make an appointment	1
2	To collect/order a repeat prescription	2
3	For treatment of an illness/condition	3
4	For a general medical examination/check-up	4
	To attend a clinic:	
5	ante-natal/pregnancy	5
6	asthma	6
7	family planning	7
8	other clinic (WRITE IN & CODE 8)	

....8

9	Blood pressure check	9
10	Cervical smear	0
11	Vaccination ('flu jab/foreign travel etc)	X
12	To get information/advice on health issues	Y

(44)

13	Family planning/contraceptive advice	1
14	Blood test	2
15	Other tests	3
16	To hear results of a test	4
17	Letter/sick note or certificate	5
18	General check of ongoing illness/condition	6
19	Letter/referral to a specialist	7
20	Other (WRITE IN & CODE 8)	

....8

None of these 9
Don't know 0

43/
44

ASK ALL WHO SAW DOCTOR/GP (CODE 1 AT Q62).　OTHERS SEE Q69 (p23)

Q65　　**How long did you have to wait at the health centre or surgery before you saw the doctor?**　WRITE IN

☐☐☐ minutes

(45)　(46)　(47)

45/
47

Q66　　**Would you say the amount of time you had to wait was ...**
READ OUT

(48)

About right 1
A little too long 2
Much too long 3
Don't know 4

48

Q67 Thinking about when you last saw your doctor/GP . . .

ASK ALL WHOSE MAIN LANGUAGE IS NOT ENGLISH AT Q21
a) In what language did you and the doctor speak to each other?

	(49)
English	1
Bengali	2
Gujerati	3
Hindi	4
Kutchi	5
Panjabi	6
Sylheti	7
Urdu	8
Other (WRITE IN & CODE '9')	
....	9
Had interpreter with me	0
Don't know	X

49

ASK ALL WHO SAW DOCTOR
b) Did the doctor give you an explanation about your condition and/or the treatment you received or not?

	(50)	
Yes, explained	1	ASK Q67c
No explanation	2	GO TO 67e
Don't know	3	
Not applicable (no explanation needed)	4	

50

ASK IF EXPLANATION GIVEN
c) Was the explanation:
READ OUT

		(51)	
	Easy to understand	1	GO TO Q67e
or	Difficult to understand	2	ASK Q67d
	Neither	3	
	Don't know	4	GO TO 67e

51

ASK IF DIFFICULT TO UNDERSTAND (CODE 2 AT Q67c)
d) Was it difficult to understand because of language problems or for other reasons? PROBE: IF OTHER: What was the reason?

	(52)
Language problems	1
Other (WRITE IN & CODE 2)	
....	2
Don't know	3

52

ASK ALL WHO SAW DOCTOR
e) Was the time the doctor spent with you . . . .
READ OUT

		(53)
	Long enough	1
or	Too short	2
	Neither	3
	Don't know	4

53

f) Did the doctor . . . .
READ OUT

(54)

Care about your
   condition/problem 1
or not care about your
   condition/problem 2
Neither 3
Don't know 4   **54**

g) Were you able to talk about the issues or problems you wanted to or not?

(55)

Yes 1
No 2
Don't know 3   **55**

h) Overall were you happy or unhappy with the outcome of your visit to the doctor?

(56)

Happy 1   ASK
Unhappy 2   Q68
Neither 3   SEE
Don't know 4   Q69   **56**

ASK IF YES
Q68   **And why was that? PROBE What else?**

. . . .

. . . .

. . . .   **57/**

. . . .   **59**

ASK ALL WHO SAW A PRACTICE NURSE (CODE 2 AT Q62). OTHERS GO TO Q70.

Q69   **Thinking about the last time you saw the practice nurse at the surgery or health centre . . .**

ASK ALL WHOSE MAIN LANGUAGE IS NOT ENGLISH AT Q21
a) In what language did you and the practice nurse speak to each other?

(60)

English 1
Bengali 2
Gujerati 3
Hindi 4
Kutchi 5
Panjabi 6
Sylheti 7
Urdu 8
Other (WRITE IN & CODE '9') . . . .

. . . . 9

Had interpreter with me 0
Don't know X   **60**

ASK ALL WHO SAW PRACTICE NURSE
b) **Did the practice nurse give you an explanation about your condition and/or the treatment you received or not?**

	(61)		
Yes, explained	1	ASK Q69c	
No explanation	2	GO TO Q70	
Don't know	3		61
Not applicable – no explanation needed	4		

ASK IF EXPLANATION GIVEN
c) **Was the explanation:**
READ OUT

		(62)		
	Easy to understand	1	GO TO Q70	
or	**Difficult to understand**	2	ASK Q69d	
	Neither	3	GO TO	
	Don't know	4	Q10	62

ASK IF DIFFICULT TO UNDERSTAND
d) **Was it difficult to understand because of language problems or for other reasons?**

	(63)	
Language problems	1	
Other (WRITE IN & CODE 2)		
....	2	
Don't know	3	63

ASK ALL

Q70 SHOWCARD Q **In the last year, which of these, if any, have you discussed with a member of staff at the surgery?**

		(64)	
1	Food that is good for your health	1	(p25)
2	Losing weight	2	(p26)
3	Exercise/fitness	3	(p27)
4	Alcohol	4	(p28)
5	Smoking	5	(p29)
6	Your worries	6	(p30)
7	Heart Disease	7	(p31)
8	Contraception/birth control	8	(p32)
9	Children's health	9	(p33)
10	Childhood Immunisation	0	(p34)
11	Cancer	X	(p35)
12	HIV/AIDS	Y	(p36)
		(65)	
13	Emotional problems (eg marital/relationship)	1	(p37)
	Other (WRITE IN & CODE 2)		
	....	2	
	Can't remember	3	
	None of these	4	GO TO Q111 (p38)

64/
65

145

1. FOOD THAT IS GOOD FOR YOU

Q71   IF NUMBER 1 AT Q70 (FOOD THAT IS GOOD FOR YOU) MENTIONED ASK:
With whom did you discuss food that is good for you? MULTICODE OK

Q72   ASK FOR EACH PERSON DISCUSSED WITH
Was it your idea to talk about food that is good for you or did ... (PERSON) start talking about it?

	Q71		Q72		
	Discussed with (66)		Resp.	Health pro	Can't remember
Doctor/GP 1			1 .... 2 3			67
Nurse....................... 2			1 .... 2 3			68
Health visitor 3			1 .... 2 3			69
Midwife 4			1 .... 2 3			70
Dietician 5			1 .... 2 3			71
Other (WRITE IN & CODE 6)					
.... 6			1 .... 2 3			72
Can't remember............. 7					

Q73   **a) Did you find the discussion on food that is good for you useful, or was it not useful?**

	(73)
Useful 1	
Not useful........................ 2	
Neither 3	
Don't know....................... 4	73

b) SHOWCARD R   Apart from discussing food that is good for you, which of these if any were you given or recommended to do?

	(74)
Asked to keep a special diary/ record sheet 1	
Given leaflets/booklets.............. 2	
Given advice on a special diet eg lactose–free, low sodium, diabetic 3	
Given a diet sheet to help you lose weight....................... 4	
Referred to a specialist/other health professional (eg dietician).......... 5	
Recommended to join a special class/ support group (eg weight watchers) .. 6	
Recommended to attend a particular clinic 7	
Take (more) exercise................ 8	
Given an exercise/fitness plan 9	
Other (WRITE IN & CODE 0)	
.... 0	
Nothing else....................... X	
Don't know....................... Y	74

2. LOSING WEIGHT

IF NUMBER 2 AT Q70 (LOSING WEIGHT) MENTIONED ASK:

Q74   **With whom did you discuss losing weight?   MULTICODE OK**

ASK FOR EACH PERSON DISCUSSED WITH

Q75   **Was it your idea to talk about losing weight or did . . . (PERSON) start talking about it?**

	Q74 Discussed with (11)	Q75 Resp.	Health pro	Can't remember	
Doctor/GP	1	1	2	3	12
Nurse.......................	2	1	2	3	13
Health visitor	3	1	2	3	14
Midwife	4	1	2	3	15
Dietician	5	1	2	3	16
Other (WRITE IN & CODE 6)					
....	6	1	2	3	17
Can't remember.............	7				

Q76   **a)   Did you find the discussion on losing weight useful, or not useful?**

	(18)	
Useful	1	
Not useful	2	
Neither	3	
Don't know.......................	4	(18)

b)   SHOWCARD S   Apart from discussing losing weight which of these, if any, were you given or recommended to do?

	(19)	
Asked to keep a special diary/ record sheet	1	
Given leaflets/booklets...............	2	
Given advice on a special diet eg lactose–free, low sodium, diabetic	3	
Given a diet sheet to help you lose weight......................	4	
Referred to a specialist/other health professional (eg dietician)..........	5	
Recommended to join a special class/ support group (eg weight watchers) ..	6	
Recommended to attend a particular clinic	7	
Take (more) exercise.................	8	
Given an exercise/fitness plan	9	
Other (WRITE IN & CODE 0)		
....	0	
Nothing else......................	X	
Don't know	Y	19

3. EXERCISE/FITNESS

IF NUMBER 3 AT Q70 (EXERCISE/FITNESS) MENTIONED ASK:

Q77 **With whom did you discuss exercise & fitness? MULTICODE OK**

ASK FOR EACH PERSON DISCUSSED WITH

Q78 **Was it your idea to talk about exercise and fitness or did . . . (PERSON) start talking about it?**

	Q77		Q78		
	Discussed with (20)	Resp.	Health pro	Can't remember	
Doctor/GP 1		1 .... 2 3			21
Nurse.......................2		1 .... 2 3			22
Health visitor 3		1 .... 2 3			23
Midwife 4		1 .... 2 3			24
Physio–therapist 5		1 .... 2 3			25
Other (WRITE IN & CODE 6)					
..........................6		1 .... 2 3			26
Can't remember..............7					

Q79 a) **Did you find the discussion on exercise and fitness useful, or not useful?**

(27)

Useful 1
Not useful.......................2
Neither 3
Don't know......................4   27

b) SHOWCARD T   **Apart from discussing exercise & fitness which of these, if any, were you given or recommended to do?**

(28)

Asked to keep a special diary/
  record sheet 1
Given leaflets/booklets..............2
Given a diet sheet 3
Referred to a specialist/other health
  professional (eg physiotherapist).....4
Recommended to join a special class/
  support group....................5
Recommended to attend a particular
  clinic..........................6
Recommended to join a special
  health/sports club 7
Exercise/fitness plan 8
Recommended to take (more)
  exercise) 9
Other (WRITE IN & CODE 0)..........0

...................................0

Nothing else.......................X
Don't know........................Y   28

4. ALCOHOL

IF NUMBER 4 AT Q70 (ALCOHOL) MENTIONED ASK:

Q80 **With whom did you discuss alcohol?** MULTICODE OK

ASK FOR EACH PERSON DISCUSSED WITH

Q81 **Was it your idea to talk about alcohol or did . . . (PERSON) start talking about it?**

	Q80		Q81		
	Discussed with (29)	Resp.	Health pro	Can't remember	
Doctor/GP 1		1	2	3	30
Nurse 2		1	2	3	31
Health visitor 3		1	2	3	32
Midwife .4		1	2	3	33
Dietician 5		1	2	3	34
Other (WRITE IN & CODE 6)					
. 6		1	2	3	35
Can't remember 7					

Q82 **a)** **Did you find the discussion on alcohol useful or not useful?**

	(36)	
Useful 1		
Not useful 2		
Neither 3		
Don't know 4		36

b) SHOWCARD U **Apart from discussing alcohol which of these if any were you given or recommended to do?**

	(37)	
Telephone a special helpline 1		
Given leaflets/booklets 2		
Referred to a specialist/other health professional 3		
Recommended to join a special class/ support group .4		
Recommended to attend a particular clinic 5		
Other (WRITE IN & CODE 6)		
. 6		
Nothing else 7		
Don't know 8		37

5. SMOKING

Q83 IF NUMBER 5 AT Q70 (SMOKING) MENTIONED ASK:
With whom did you discuss smoking? MULTICODE OK

Q84 ASK FOR EACH PERSON DISCUSSED WITH
Was it your idea to start talking about smoking or did . . . (PERSON) start talking about it?

	Q83		Q84	
	Discussed with (38)	Resp.	Health pro	Can't remember
Doctor/GP 1		1 ....2 3			39
Nurse......................2		1 ....2 3			40
Health visitor 3		1 ....2 3			41
Midwife 4		1 ....2 3			42
Dietician 5		1 ....2 3			43
Other (WRITE IN & CODE 6)					
..........................6		1 ....2 3			44
Can't remember..............7					

Q85 **a) Did you find the discussion on smoking useful, or not useful?**

(45)
Useful 1
Not useful 2
Neither 3
Don't know 4   45

b) SHOWCARD V Apart from discussing smoking which of these if any were you given or recommended to do?

(46)
Asked to keep a special diary/
    record sheet 1
Given leaflets/booklets...............2
Referred to a specialist/other health
    professional......................3
Recommended to join a special class/
    support group....................4
Recommended to attend a particular
    smoking clinic 5
Telephone a special helpline 6
Recommended to take nicotine
    substitutes 7
Other (WRITE IN & CODE 8) ....
..........................8
Nothing else.....................9
Don't know 0   46

6. YOUR WORRIES

Q86 IF NUMBER 6 AT Q70 (WORRIES) MENTIONED ASK:
With whom did you discuss your worries? MULTICODE OK

Q87 ASK FOR EACH PERSON DISCUSSED WITH
Was it your idea to start talking about your worries or did . . . (PERSON) start talking about it?

	Q86 Discussed with (47)	Q87 Resp.	Health pro	Can't remember	
Doctor/GP	1	1	2	3	48
Nurse......................	2	1	2	3	49
Health visitor	3	1	2	3	50
Midwife	4	1	2	3	51
Councellor	5	1	2	3	52
Social worker	6	1	2	3	53
Other (WRITE IN & CODE 7)					
....	7	1	2	3	54
Can't remember..............	8				

Thinking about the discussion on your worries

Q88 a) **Did you find the discussion on your worries useful, or not useful?**

(55)
Useful 1
Not useful 2
Neither 3
Don't know....................... 4   55

b) **SHOWCARD W   Apart from discussing your worries which of these if any were you given or recommended to do?**

(56)
Asked to keep a special diary/
   record sheet 1
Given leaflets/booklets............... 2
Referred to a specialist/other health
   professional 3
Recommended to join a special class/
   support group 4
Recommended to attend a particular
   clinic (eg stress clinic) 5
Recommended to take exercise 6
Other (WRITE IN & CODE 7) ....

   7

Nothing else....................... 8
Don't know....................... 9   56

7. HEART DISEASE

Q89   IF NUMBER 7 AT Q70 (HEART DISEASE) MENTIONED ASK:
With whom did you discuss heart disease? MULTICODE OK

Q90   ASK FOR EACH PERSON DISCUSSED WITH
Was it your idea to start talking about heart disease, or did . . . (PERSON) start talking about it?

	Q89		Q90		
	Discussed with (57)	Resp.	Health pro	Can't remember	
Doctor/GP 1		1 . . . . 2 3			58
Nurse. .2		1 . . . . 2 3			59
Health visitor 3		1 . . . . 2 3			60
Midwife 4		1 . . . . 2 3			61
Dietician 5		1 . . . . 2 3			62
Other (WRITE IN & CODE 6)					
. 6		1 . . . . 2 3			63
Can't remember 7					

Q91   **a) Did you find the discussion on heart disease useful, or not useful?**

	(64)	
Useful 1		
Not useful 2		
Neither 3		
Don't know 4		64

b) SHOWCARD X   Apart from discussing heart disease which of these if any were you given or recommended to do?

	(65)	
Asked to keep a special diary/ record sheet 1		
Given leaflets/booklets 2		
Given a diet sheet 3		
Referred to a specialist/other health professional 4		
Recommended to join a special class/ support group 5		
Recommended to attend a particular clinic 6		
Take (more) exercise 7		
Reduce weight 8		
Reduce smoking 9		
Other (WRITE IN & CODE 0)		
. 0		
Nothing else X		
Don't know . . . . .Y		65

8. CONTRACEPTION/BIRTH CONTROL

Q92
IF NUMBER 8 AT Q70 (CONTRACEPTION/BIRTH CONTROL) MENTIONED ASK:
With whom did you discuss contraception/birth control? MULTICODE OK

Q93
ASK FOR EACH PERSON DISCUSSED WITH
And was it your idea to start talking about contraception/birth control, or did ... (PERSON) start talking about it?

	Q92 Discussed with (66)		Q93 Resp.	Health pro	Can't remember	
Doctor/GP	1		1	2	3	67
Nurse	2		1	2	3	68
Health visitor	3		1	2	3	69
Midwife	4		1	2	3	70
Dietician	5		1	2	3	71
Other (WRITE IN & CODE 6)						
....	6		1	2	3	72
Can't remember	7					

Q94
a) Did you find the discussion on contraception/birth control useful, or not useful?

	(73)	
Useful	1	
Not useful	2	
Neither	3	
Don't know	4	73

b) SHOWCARD Y   Apart from discussing contraception/birth control which of these, if any, were you given or recommended to do?

	(74)	
Asked to keep a special diary/ temperature chart	1	
Given leaflets/booklets	2	
Given free condoms	3	
Referred to a specialist/other health professional	4	
Recommended to attend a particular clinic (eg Family Planning)	5	
Other (WRITE IN & CODE 6)		
....	6	
Nothing else	7	
Don't know	8	74

CARD 6   10

9. CHILDREN'S HEALTH

Q95   IF NUMBER 9 AT Q70 (CHILDREN'S HEALTH) MENTIONED ASK:
       With whom did you discuss children's health? MULTICODE OK

       ASK FOR EACH PERSON DISCUSSED WITH
Q95   **And was it your idea to start talking about children's health or did . . . (PERSON)
       start talking about it?**

	Q95			Q96		
	Discussed with (11)		Resp.	Health pro	Can't remember	
Doctor/GP 1			1 .... 2 3			12
Nurse 2			1 .... 2 3			13
Health visitor 3			1 .... 2 3			14
Midwife 4			1 .... 2 3			15
Dietician 5			1 .... 2 3			16
Other (WRITE IN & CODE 6)						
.... 6			1 .... 2 3			17
Can't remember 7						

Q97   **Did you find the discussion on children's health useful, or not useful?**

                                                    (18)
            Useful 1
            Not useful 2
            Neither 3
            Don't know 4   18

10. CHILDHOOD IMMUNISATION

IF NUMBER 10 AT Q70 (CHILDHOOD IMMUNISATION) MENTIONED ASK:

Q98 **With whom did you discuss childhood immunisation?** MULTICODE OK

ASK FOR EACH PERSON DISCUSSED WITH

Q99 **Was it your idea to start talking about childhood immunisation, or did . . . (PERSON) start talking about it?**

	Q98 Discussed with (19)		Q99 Resp.	Health pro	Can't remember	
Doctor/GP	1		1	2	3	20
Nurse	2		1	2	3	21
Health visitor	3		1	2	3	22
Midwife	4		1	2	3	23
Other (WRITE IN & CODE 5)						
	5		1	2	3	24
Can't remember	6					

Q100 **a) Did you find the discussion on childhood immunisation useful, or not useful?**

	(25)	
Useful	1	
Not useful	2	
Neither	3	
Don't know	4	25

b) SHOWCARD Z **Apart from discussing childhood immunisation which of these if any were you given or recommended to do?**

	(26)	
Given leaflets/booklets	1	
Referred to a specialist/other health professional	2	
Recommended to attend a particular clinic (eg immunisation clinic)	3	
Other (WRITE IN & CODE 4)		
	4	
Nothing else	5	
Don't know	6	26

155

11. CANCER

Q101
IF NUMBER 11 AT Q70 (CANCER) MENTIONED ASK:
With whom did you discuss cancer? MULTICODE OK

Q102
ASK FOR EACH PERSON DISCUSSED WITH
Was it your idea to start talking about cancer or did . . . (PERSON) start talking about it?

	Q101 Discussed with (27)	Resp.	Q102 Health pro	Can't remember	
Doctor/GP 1		1 .... 2 3			28
Nurse 2		1 .... 2 3			29
Health visitor 3		1 .... 2 3			30
Midwife 4		1 .... 2 3			31
Dietician 5		1 .... 2 3			32
Other (WRITE IN & CODE 6)					
.... 6		1 .... 2 3			33
Can't remember 7					

Q104 **a) Did you find the discussion on cancer useful, or not useful?**

	(34)	
Useful 1		
Not useful 2		
Neither 3		
Don't know 4		34

b) SHOWCARD AA   Apart from discussing cancer which of these if any were you given or recommended to do?

	(35)	
Asked to keep a special diary/ record sheet 1		
Given leaflets/booklets 2		
Given a diet sheet 3		
Referred to a specialist/other health professional 4		
Recommended to join a special class/ support group 5		
Recommended to attend a particular clinic 6		
Recommended to a counsellor 7		
Recommended to contact specialist/cancer organisation/ charity............................ 8		
Other (WRITE IN & CODE 9)		
.... 9		
Nothing else 0		
Don't know X		35

12. HIV/AIDS

Q105
IF NUMBER 12 AT Q70 (HIV/AIDS) MENTIONED ASK:
With whom did you discuss HIV/AIDS? MULTICODE OK

Q106
ASK FOR EACH PERSON DISCUSSED WITH
Was it your idea to start talking about HIV/AIDS, or did . . . (PERSON) start talking about it?

	Q105 Discussed with (36)	Resp.	Q106 Health pro	Can't remember	
Doctor/GP	1	1	2	3	37
Nurse	2	1	2	3	38
Health visitor	3	1	2	3	39
Midwife	4	1	2	3	40
Counsellor	5	1	2	3	41
Social Worker	6	1	2	3	42
Other (WRITE IN & CODE 7)					
	7	1	2	3	43
Can't remember	8				

Q107 a) **Did you find the discussion on HIV/AIDS useful, or not useful**

	(44)	
Useful	1	
Not useful	2	
Neither	3	
Don't know	4	44

b) **SHOWCARD BB   Apart from discussing HIV/AIDS which of these, if any, were you given or recommended to do?**

	(45)	
Given leaflets/booklets	1	
Referred to a specialist/other health professional	2	
Recommended to join a special class/ support group	3	
Recommended to attend a particular clinic	4	
Recommended to see a counsellor	5	
Recommended to contact specialist HIV/AIDs organisation or charity	6	
Given needles	7	
Given condoms	8	
Other (WRITE IN & CODE 9)		
	9	
Nothing else	0	
Don't know	X	45

13. EMOTIONAL PROBLEMS

Q108   IF NUMBER 13 AT Q70 (EMOTIONAL PROBLEMS) MENTIONED ASK:
With whom did you discuss emotional problems? MULTICODE OK

Q109   ASK FOR EACH PERSON DISCUSSED WITH
Was it your idea to start talking about emotional problems, or did . . . (PERSON) start talking about it?

	Q108 Discussed with (46)		Resp.	Q109 Health pro	Can't remember	
Doctor/GP	1		1	2	3	47
Nurse	2		1	2	3	48
Health visitor	3		1	2	3	49
Midwife	4		1	2	3	50
Councellor	5		1	2	3	51
Social worker	6		1	2	3	52
Other (WRITE IN & CODE 6)						
....	7		1	2	3	53
Can't remember	8					

Q110   a) **Did you find the discussion about emotional problems useful, or not useful?**

(54)
Useful 1
Not useful 2
Neither 3
Don't know 4   (54)

     b) SHOWCARD CC   **Apart from discussing emotional problems which of these if any were you given or recommended to do?**

(55)
Asked to keep a special diary/
     record sheet 1
Given leaflets/booklets 2
Referred to a specialist/other health
     professional 3
Recommended to join a special class/
     support group 4
Recommended to attend a particular
     clinic 5
Recommended to see a counsellor 6
Recommended to contact specialist
     organisation/charity 7
Other (WRITE IN & CODE 8)

     8

Nothing else 9
Don't know 0   55

ASK ALL
Q111 SHOWCARD DD   Looking at this card, could you tell me please which, if any, of these you have used in the last 12 months?

(56)

1   Family planning clinic....................................1
2   Community midwife..2
3   Health visitor 3
4   Chiropodist..4
5   District nurse 5
6   Optician 6
7   Chiropractor...7
8   Acupuncturist 8
9   Homeopath 9
10 Osteopath 0
11 Aromatherapist X
12 Dentist ....Y

(57)

13 Hakims/Vaid 1
14 Aruiis 2
15 Mataji's 3
    Other (WRITE IN AND CODE 4) ....

   4
    Can't remember 5   56/
    None of these 6   57

Q112   SHOWCARD EE   What subjects dealing with your health or being healthy would you like information or more information about? PROBE: What else?
DO NOT PROMPT

(58)

Physical exercise 1
Healthy eating.......................2
Stopping smoking 3
Children's health 4
HIV/AIDS 5
Sexually transmitted
  disease 6
Advice on contraception/
  family planning 7
Drinking alcohol 8
Drugs 9
Heart disease/
  heart attacks 0
Menstruation/periods X
Sex education.......................Y

(59)

Coping with worries/pressures 1
Other (WRITE IN AND CODE 2).......2

....
Nothing 3   58/
Don't know 4   59

159

Q113 SHOWCARD FF   How easy or difficult would you find it to discuss each of the following issues with your GP or another health professional at the surgery or health centre? READ OUT. ROTATE ORDER. TICK START

		1 Very easy	2 Fairly easy	3 Fairly difficult	4 Very Difficult	5 No opinion	6 Don't know	
a	Weight control	1	2	3	4	5	6	60
b	Alcohol	1	2	3	4	5	6	61
c	Smoking	1	2	3	4	5	6	62
d	Stress	1	2	3	4	5	6	63
e	Contraception/birth control	1	2	3	4	5	6	64
f	Children's health	1	2	3	4	5	6	65
g	HIV/AIDS	1	2	3	4	5	6	66
h	Mental or psychological problems (eg. depression, anxiety)	1	2	3	4	5	6	67
i	Emotional problems (eg marital/ relationship)	1	2	3	4	5	6
j	Sexual problems (eg sexually transmitted diseases)	1	2	3	4	5	6	69

ASK WOMEN ONLY

k	Gynaecological problems (eg period problems, infections such as thrush etc)	1	2	3	4	5	6	70

ASK ALL

Q114 SHOWCARD GG   Thinking about different ways you can get advice on health matters, which of these have you ever used?

(71)

Leaflets from your GP 1
Leaflets in shop/supermarkets 2
Advice from your GP or community worker..... 3
Video for use at home 4
Television programme 5
Information in magazines 6
Information in local/community newspapers ... 7
Information in National newspapers.......... 8
National radio.............................. 9
Local/community radio 0
Other (WRITE IN AND CODE X) ....

.... X

None..................................... Y

(72)

Don't know 1

71/
72

Q115 **In which language would you prefer to listen to health advice on the TV or Radio?**
MULTICODE OK

	(73)
English...	1
Bengall	2
Gujeratl	3
Hindl	4
Panjabl	5
Sylhetl	6
Urdu..	7
Other (WRITE IN & CODE 8)	
....	8
Don't know	9

73

ASK ALL EXCEPT THOSE UNABLE TO READ ANY LANGUAGE (CODE 9, Q20, p4)
Q116 **In what language would you prefer to read about health advice?**
MULTICODE OK

	(74)
English...	1
Bengall	2
Gujeratl	3
Hindl	4
Panjabl (Urdu or Perso–Arabic Script)	5
Panjabl (Sikh or Gurmukhi Script)	6
Urdu..	7
Other (WRITE IN & CODE 8)	
....	8
Don't know	9

74

CANCER SCREENING

ASK ALL

Q117 **I'd now like to ask you a few questions about medical examination (that is the taking of a sample for tests). Have you ever had an examination for any type of cancer?** IF YES: **What type of cancer?** CODE BELOW

ASK FOR EACH ONE MENTIONED

Q118 **Was the examination for . . . (TYPE OF CANCER) carried out on the NHS or privately?**

	Q117		Q118		
Yes:			NHS	Private	Don't know
	(75)					
Breast cancer 1			1 .... 2 3			76
Cervical smear 2			1 .... 2 3			77
Skin cancer 3	ASK Q126		1 .... 2 3			78
Testicular cancer 4			1 .... 2 3			79
Lung cancer..................... 5					
Other (WRITE IN & CODE 5).........					
.... 6			1 .... 2 3			80
No, never had examination 7					
Don't know 8	SEE Q127				
Refused 9					

CARD 7   10

ASK WOMEN ONLY. MEN GO TO Q122

Q119 **Have you ever had a cervical smear test (when they take a sample of cells from the neck of the womb or uterus)?** IF YES **When did you last have a smear test?**

(11)
In last week............................ 1
Within last 6 months 2
Over 6 months, within last 12 months 3
Over 1 year, within last 3 years............ 4
Over 3 years, within last 5 years............ 5
Over 5 years 6
Can't remember 7
Never 8   11

Q120 **In the last 12 months, has any health professional <u>suggested</u> you consider having a smear test, or given you an appointment or a written invitation to have a cervical smear test?**

(12)
Yes 1
No/don't know 2   12

ASK IF NEVER HAD SMEAR TEST AT Q119. OTHERS GO TO Q122

Q121 **Why have you never had a smear test?**

(13)
Never been sexually active.................. 1
Never been told/recommended to 2
Embarrassment 3
Scared 4
Doesn't do any good 5
Rather not know 6
Don't think I need one 7
Too busy/never got round to it 8
Other (WRITE IN & CODE 9) ....
.... 9
Don't know what smear test is 0
Don't know X   13

SMOKING

ASK ALL
Q122 I would now like to ask you a few questions about smoking. Whilst I am aware smoking may be offensive to you and against your religion please understand it is important we ask everyone this question. Have you ever smoked a cigarette, cigar or pipe?

(14)

Yes 1   ASK Q123

No...................................... 2   GO TO Q149 (p47)   14

ASK ALL WHO EVER SMOKED. OTHERS GO TO Q149 (p47)
Q123 Do you smoke cigarettes at all nowadays?

(15)

Yes 1   GO TO Q132 (p44)

No...................................... 2   ASK Q124   15

ASK EX–CIGARETTE SMOKERS. OTHERS GO TO Q132 (p44)
Q124 Have you ever smoked cigarettes regularly?

(16)

Yes 1   ASK Q125

No...................................... 2   GO TO Q149 (p47)   16

ASK EX–REGULAR SMOKERS (YES AT Q124). OTHERS GO TO Q149 (p47)
Q125 How old were you when you first tried smoking?

☐☐ years

(17) (18)   17/
18

Q126 And how old were you when you started to smoke regularly?

☐☐ years

(19) (20)   19/
20

Q127 How many cigarettes did you smoke in a day when you were a regular smoker?

☐☐☐ cigarettes a day

(21) (22) (23)   21/
23

ROLL–UPS ☐☐ grammes of tobacco

(24) (25)   24/
25

Q128 How long ago did you give up smoking?

(26)

In last 6 months........................... 1
In last 12 months.......................... 2
In last 2 years............................ 3
In last 5 years............................ 4
In last 10 years........................... 5
Longer ago 6
Can't remember 7   26

Q129 Why did you give up smoking? PROBE FULLY. MULTICODE OK

                                               (27)

Diagnosis of health problems 1   GO
Advice from doctor (but no diagnosis   TO
    of health problems) 2   Q131
Pregnancy 3
Cost/save money 4
General concern about health/fitness 5
Became more aware of health risks
    of smoking (eg read something) 6   SEE
Pressure from family 7   Q130
Aesthetic/cosmetic reasons, eg. smell,
    yellow teeth, nicotine stains 8
Pressure from friends/work colleagues 9
Set example for family 0
Worried about effects of passive smoking
    on family X
Because people can't smoke at work .... Y
                                               (28)
Recommended by doctor 1
No specific reason 2
Other (WRITE IN & CODE '3') ....

.... 3   27/
Don't know 4   28

ASK IF CODES 1–3 NOT MENTIONED AT Q129

Q130 Did anything in particular happen to make you want to give up at that time? IF YES: What was this?

                                             (29)

No, nothing 1

Yes:

New Year's Resolution 2
Advertising campaign 3
TV programme 4
No Smoking Day 5
No smoking policy at work 6
Smoking–related illness/death
    of relative/friend 7
Cost of cigarettes went up/tax on
    tobacco increased/budget day 8
Talked to smoking advice/
    counselling phone line 9
Other (WRITE IN & CODE 0) ....

.... 0

Don't know X   29

ASK ALL EX-REGULAR SMOKERS

Q131 About how many times did you attempt to give up smoking before you succeeded?

                                             (30)

Succeeded first time 1
Twice 2
3–4 times 3
5–9 times 4   NOW GO TO Q149 (p47)
10–14 times 5
15–19 times 6
20+ times 7
Can't remember 8   30

ASK CURRENT SMOKERS ONLY (YES AT Q123). OTHERS GO TO Q149 (p47)
Q132 **Do you smoke cigarettes regularly nowadays?**

(31)
Yes 1   ASK Q133
No.. 2   GO TO Q149 (p47)   31

Q133 **How old were you when you first tried smoking?**

☐☐ years

(32) (33)   32/
                                                                                 33

Q134 **And how old were you when you started to smoke regularly?**

☐☐ years

(34) (35)   34/
                                                                                 35

Q135 **How many cigarettes do you smoke in an average day?**

☐☐☐ cigarettes

(36) (37) (38)   36/
                                                                                 38

ROLL–UPS   ☐☐ grammes of tobacco   39
(39) (40)   40

Q136 **Did you smoke any cigarettes yesterday?**

(41)
Yes 1   ASK Q137
No.. 2   GO TO Q138   41

Q137 **How many cigarettes did you smoke yesterday?**

☐☐☐ cigarettes
(42) (43) (44)   42/44

NB. IF "ROLL YOUR OWN" GIVE AMOUNT OF TOBACCO USED

☐☐ grammes
(45) (46)   45/46

ASK ALL CURRENT REGULAR SMOKERS (YES AT Q123)
Q138 **Do you ever smoke in your own home, or not?**

(47)
Yes 1
No 2   47

Q139 **Do you want to continue being a smoker or do you want to give up smoking?**

(48)
Continue 1   GO TO Q141
Give up 2   ASK Q140
Don't know 3   GO TO Q141   48

ASK IF WANT TO GIVE UP AT Q139
Q140 **Do you have any firm plans to give up smoking in the future, or not?**

	(49)	
Yes	1	
No/not sure	2	**49**

ASK ALL CURRENT REGULAR SMOKERS
Q141 **Have you ever tried to give up smoking?**

	(50)	
Yes	1	ASK Q142
No...	2	GO TO Q145 (p46)	**50**

ASK THOSE WHO HAVE TRIED TO GIVE UP (YES AT Q141). OTHERS GO TO Q145
Q142 **About how many times have you tried to give up smoking?**

	(51)	
Once	1	
Twice	2	
3–4 times	3	
5–9 times	4	
10–14 times	5	
15–19 times	6	
20+ times	7	
Can't remember	8	**51**

Q143 **What factors or events made you take up smoking again? MULTICODE OK**

	(52)	
Weight gain	1	
Worries	2	
Lack of will–power	3	
Encouragement by friends/colleagues/ peer group pressure	4	
Encouragement by family members	5	
Withdrawal symptoms, eg. headaches shakes, irritability	6	
Loss of enjoyment	7	
Loss of social prop/need something to do with hands.........................	8	
Other (WRITE IN & CODE 9)		
....	9	
Nothing in particular.......................	0	
Don't know	X	**52**

Q144 SHOWCARD HH   Here is a list of things some people have used to give up smoking. Could you tell me please which, if any, you have used? MULTICODE OK

		Used
		(53)
1	Help and support from family	1
2	Help and support from friends	2
3	Help and support at work	3
4	Advice and support from doctor.....................	4
5	Prescription from doctor............................	5
6	Aids bought from chemist (eg. nicorettes)...........	6
7	Special clinics or 'stop smoking' groups	7
8	Booklets with advice and practical tips on how to stop smoking	8
9	Individual counselling and advice	9
10	Quitline/telephone helpline/ advice line........................	0
11	"How to quit" videos	X
12	Alternative treatments such as hypnosis or acupuncture	Y

	(54)
Other (PLEASE SPECIFY & CODE 1)	
.... 1	
None of these 2	53/
Don't know 3	54

ASK ALL CURRENT REGULAR SMOKERS (YES AT Q123)
Q145 SHOWCARD II   How much, if at all, do you think the amount you smoke affects your health now?

	(55)	
A great deal........................ 1		
A fair amount 2		
Just a little 3	ASK Q146	
Not at all 4	GO TO	
Don't know......................... 5	Q147	(55)

ASK IF CODES 1–3 AT Q145. OTHERS GO TO Q147
Q146 In what ways do you think it affects your health now? PROBE: What others?

	(56)	
Breathlessness 1		
Coughing 2		
Wheezing 3		
Prone to chest infections..................... 4		
Less fit than I used to be..................... 5		
Worry about serious illnesses................. 6		
Other (WRITE IN & CODE 7)....................		
.... 7		
Don't know............................... 8	56	

ASK ALL CURRENT REGULAR SMOKERS

Q147 SHOWCARD II AGAIN   And how much, if at all, do you think the amount you smoke will affect your health in the future?

```
                                                            (57)
        A great deal ................................... 1
        A fair amount .................................. 2
        Just a little .................................... 3    ASK Q148
        Not at all ...................................... 4    GO TO
        Don't know ..................................... 5    Q149              57
```

ASK IF CODES 1-3 AT Q147

Q148 In what ways do you think it will affect your health in the future? PROBE: What others?

```
                                                            (58)
        Likely to get heart disease ................... 1
        Likely to get chest infections/bronchitis ....... 2
        Likely to get lung cancer ..................... 3
        Likely to get other cancer .................... 4
        Likely to get cancer (unspecified) ............ 5
        Likely to get lung problems (unspecified) ....... 6
        Likely to get problems with breathing/
          coughing/wheezing ......................... 7
        Likely to get breathlessness .................. 8
        Likely to become less fit ..................... 9
        Likely to get a serious illness (unspecified) ..... 0
        Other (WRITE IN & CODE X) ..................

        ...........................................X

        Don't know .............................. Y            58
```

ASK ALL

Q149 In an average day, do you spend any time in places where you are inhaling other people's cigarette smoke, or not?

```
                              (59)
        Yes ..................... 1   ASK Q150
        No...................... 2   SEE Q152
        Don't know ............. 3                            59
```

ASK IF YES AT Q149

Q150 In an average day, would you spend any time exposed to other people's cigarette smoke ... READ OUT AND CODE A RESPONSE ON EACH ITEM

	Yes	No	Don't know	Not applicable	
at home	1	2	3	4	60
at work	1	2	3	4	61
in shops	1	2	3	4	62
in pubs or restaurants	1	2	3	4	63
in other places you go socially	1	2	3	4	64
while travelling	1	2	3	4	65

Q151 And how much time would you say you spend in an average day, in places where you are inhaling other people's cigarette smoke?

☐☐ hours   ☐☐ minutes

(66) (67)   (68) (69)

66/
69

(70)
Don't know .... Y

70

IF RESPONDENT IS CODED 1 OR 2 AT Q28 P6 (WORKING BUT NOT SELF-EMPLOYED), ASK Q152. OTHERS GO TO Q153.

Q152 SHOWCARD JJ   Which, if any, of these does your employer do about smoking at work? MULTICODE OK

(71)

01	Leaflets on how to stop smoking 1
02	Posters on how to stop smoking...................... 2
03	There are no restrictions on smoking at work 3
04	Smoking is allowed in private offices only 4
05	Smoking is allowed in catering/eating area only 5
06	Smoking is allowed in customer/visitor area only 6
07	A complete ban on smoking at work 3
08	No smoking signs 4
09	A smoking room 5
10	Advice from works doctor/nurse..................... 6
11	Advice from personnel officers 7
12	Advice from outside counsellors 8
13	Work with trade unions to promote smoking bans/control.................. 9
14	Contact with self-help groups (eg stop smoking groups) 0
15	Run stop smoking groups X
16	Support from management to reduce work stress .... Y

(72)

17	Time off for counselling or treatment 1
	Other (WRITE IN & CODE '2') ....
	 2
	None of these 3
	Don't know 4

71/
72

ASK ALL
Q153 SHOWCARD KK   Which, if any, of these have you ever used?

Q154 SHOWCARD KK AGAIN   And which, if any, do you use nowadays? CODE BELOW

	Q153 (73)	Q154 (74)
Betel nut/Sopari chewed with tobacco	1	1
Betel nut/Sopari chewed with no tobacco	2	2
Chewing tobacco	3	3
Paan	4	4
Hukka	5	5
Bidi...................................	6	6
Other tobacco substance (WRITE IN & CODE 7)		
....	7	7
None of these...........................	8 GO TO	8
Don't know	9 Q155	9

73/
74

ONLY ASK Q155 AND Q156 IF RESPONDENT IS HEAD OF HOUSEHOLD
I would now just like to ask you some questions about the people in your
household. These questions are personal but no one will be able to identify
individual households. It is important we ask these questions so that we can
assess the needs of different groups of people.

Q155a Respondent Head of Household?

```
                                                      (75)
Yes ....................................... 1    ASK Q155b
No........................................ 2    GO TO READ
                                                 OUT BEFORE Q157         75
```

**Q155b SHOWCARD LL   Do you receive any of these benefits, either for yourself or on
behalf of the household?**

```
                                                          (76)
Child benefit.................................................1
State retirement pension ...............................2
Income Support/social security .....................3
Unemployment benefit ...................................4
Family Credit .................................................5
Housing Benefit .............................................6
Attendance Allowance ...................................7
Invalid Care Allowance .................................8
Mobility Allowance ........................................9
Sickness Benefit ...........................................0
Disablement living allowance ........................ X
Other (WRITE IN & CODE Y) ...........................

...................................................................... Y
                                                          (77)            76/
None of these..............................................1            77
```

Q156   SHOWCARD MM   Household Income
Could you please give me the letter from this card for the group in which you
would place your total household income from all sources, <u>before</u> tax and other
deductions?

Please include all benefits, such as child benefit, Income Support, retirement
pensions, unemployment benefit. Please also remember to include income from
all members of the household.

```
                                              (78)
A.................................................. 1
B.................................................. 2
C.................................................. 3
D.................................................. 4
E.................................................. 5
F.................................................. 6
G.................................................. 7
H.................................................. 8
I.................................................. 9
J.................................................. 0
K.................................................. X
L.................................................. Y
                                              (79)
M .................................................. 1
Don't know ..................................... 2            78/
Refused .......................................... 3            79
```

INTERVIEWER: IF DEMOGRAPHICS NOT ALREADY COMPLETED, DO THESE NOW. THEN CHECK FOR LITERACY IN ENGLISH OR OTHER SURVEY LANGUAGE (CODE 1, 2, 3, 6 OR 7 AT Q20 P4). IF LITERATE IN SURVEY LANGUAGE, HAND OVER SELF-COMPLETION QUESTIONNAIRE, CHECKING FOR MEN'S/WOMEN'S VERSION. **DO <u>NOT</u> GIVE THE QUESTIONNAIRE TO RESPONDENTS AGED 55+ (THESE RESPONDENTS GO STRAIGHT TO Q157).**
IF NOT LITERATE IN SURVEY LANGUAGE GO STRAIGHT TO Q157.

CARD 8	10

SAY "This questionnaire is designed for you to complete on your own. Please read the instructions on the front page carefully and then try to answer the questions.

I realise you may consider some of these questions very personal. They may concern matters that normally you do not discuss even with your partner or close friends. However, if we are to provide relevant health care for the Asian community it is essential that we have more information on these matters.

STRESS:

- ENTIRELY PRIVATE: NO NAME ON QUESTIONNAIRE AND INTERVIEWER WILL NOT SEE ANSWERS

- SERIOUS PIECE OF MEDICAL/SOCIAL RESEARCH

- SURVEY ALREADY COMPLETED AMONGST GENERAL POPULATION, NEED INFORMATION FROM ASIAN COMMUNITY FOR COMPARISON PURPOSES

When you have finished put the questionnaire into the brown envelope, seal it and hand it back to me.

THEN WHEN SELF-COMPLETION QUESTIONNAIRE DONE COME BACK TO Q157.

CODE RESPONSE TO SELF-COMPLETION

(11)
Questionnaire accepted 1
Questionnaire refused 2
Questionnaire not handed over because
  respondent aged 55+ 3
Questionnaire not handed over because
  respondent not literate in survey languages 4

11

Q157 We have almost come to the end of the questionnaire now, in which we have covered a number of different health issues. Are there any other health concerns you have which have not been covered? IF YES, PROBE. And what concerns have not been covered? PROBE FULLY

(12)
No additional concerns 1
Additional concerns (WRITE IN
  & CODE 2) 2

....

....

....

....

12/
15

Respondent Feedback

I would like to end the interview by asking you what you thought about the interview.

Q158 How interesting did you find the interview? Would you say ...
READ OUT. ALTERNATE & TICK START

(16)
☐ ... very interesting 1
... fairly interesting 2
... not very interesting 3
☐ ... not at all interesting 4
Don't know 5   16

Q159 Were there any sections which you found difficult to answer?

(17)
Yes 1
No 2   17

Q160 And how long did you find the interview? Would you say ...
READ OUT. ALTERNATE & TICK START

(18)
☐ ... much too long 1
... a little too long 2
... about right 3
☐ ... too short 4
Don't know 5   18

Q161 Did you think the questions were difficult to understand or not? Would you say they were ...
READ OUT. ALTERNATE & TICK START

(19)
☐ ... very difficult 1
... fairly difficult 2
... not very difficult 3
☐ ... not at all difficult 4
Don't know 5   19

Q162 Finally, how interested would you be in participating in future surveys on similar subjects? Would you be ...
READ OUT. ALTERNATE & TICK START

(20)
☐ ... very interested 1
... fairly interested 2
... not very interested 3
☐ ... not at all interested 4
Don't know 5   20

INTERVIEWER CODE:

This interview was carried out:

                                                   (21)

    In total privacy throughout 1
    With someone else present for part of
      the interview 2
    With someone else present for most of/
      all of the interview 3   **21**

IF SOMEONE ELSE WAS PRESENT (CODES 2 OR 3)

The other person/people present was/were:

                                                     (22)

    Respondent's spouse/partner 1
    Respondent's child/ren 2
    Respondent's parent/s or other relatives 3
    Other 4
    Don't know 5   **22**

INTERVIEWER ASSESSMENT:

This respondent's level of literacy seemed:

                                                     (23)

    Good 1
    Average 2
    Poor 3   **23**

Length of interview write in   ☐☐☐ minutes   **24/ 26**

                    (24) (25) (26)

THANK RESPONDENT & CLOSE

173